ANATOMY
And
PHYSIOLOGY

coloring and activity book

Med Dani coloring

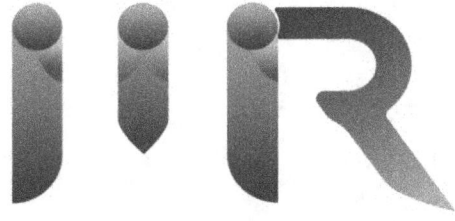

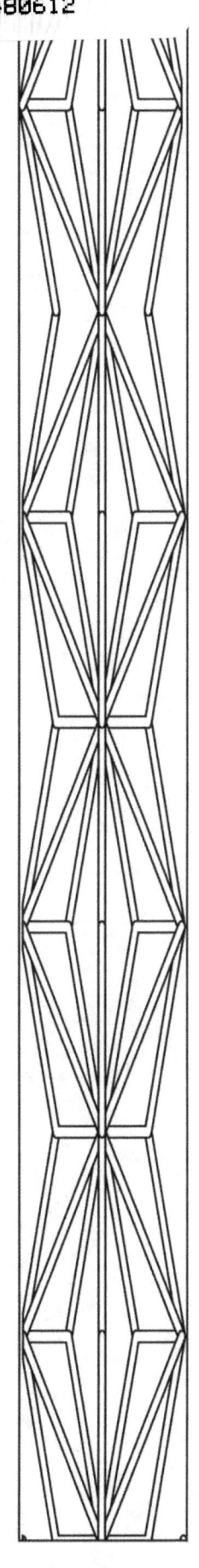
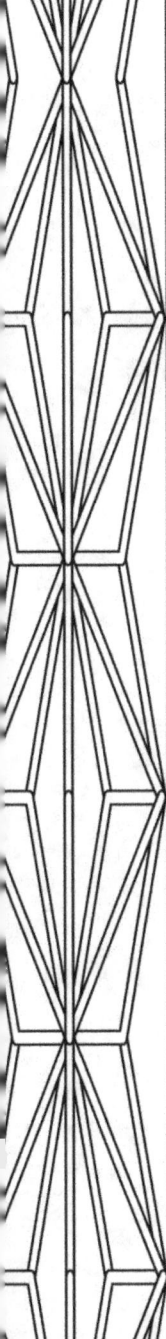

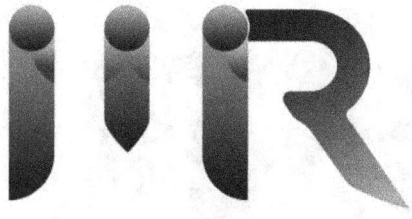

CONTENTS

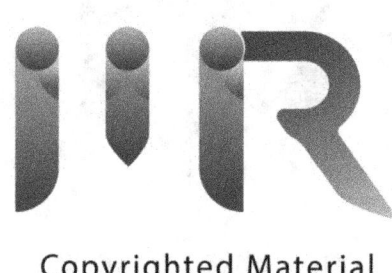

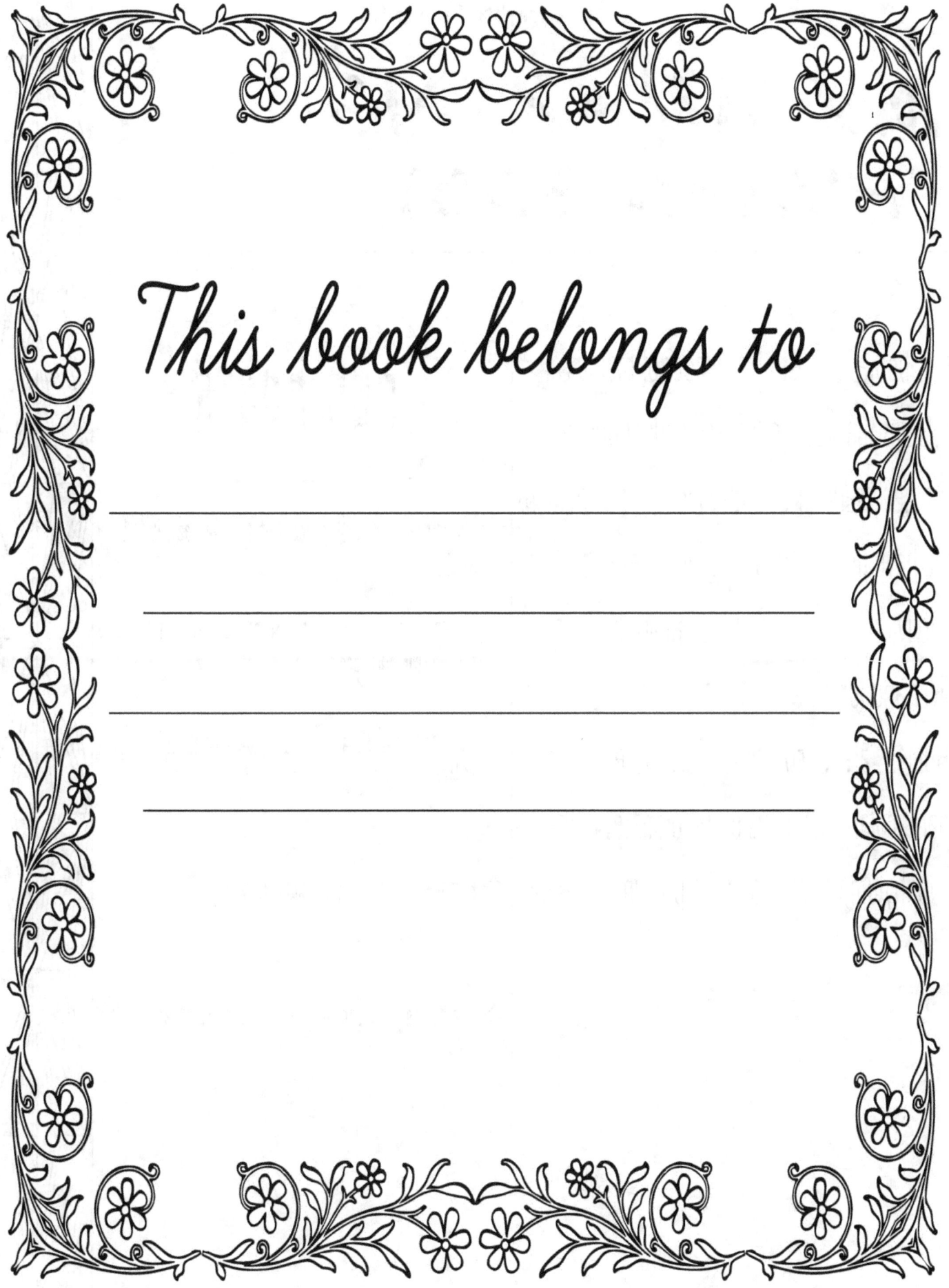

This book belongs to

MY AMAZING HUMAN BODY

Our bodies consist of a number of biological systems that carry out specific functions that are necessary for everyday living. Us as humans we have five vital organs that are essential for survival. These are the brain, heart, kidneys, liver and lungs.

Humans are, of course animals_more pareticulary, members of the primates in the subphylum vertebrata of the phylum chordata.

Fun Facts

✧ Water makes up to 50 percent of the average adults body weight.

✧ During you're life time, you will produce enough saliva to fill two swimmings pools.

✧ Your nose and ears continue growing throughout your entire life.

✧ Humans are the only animals with chins.

✧ The human body contains enough to make seven bars of soap

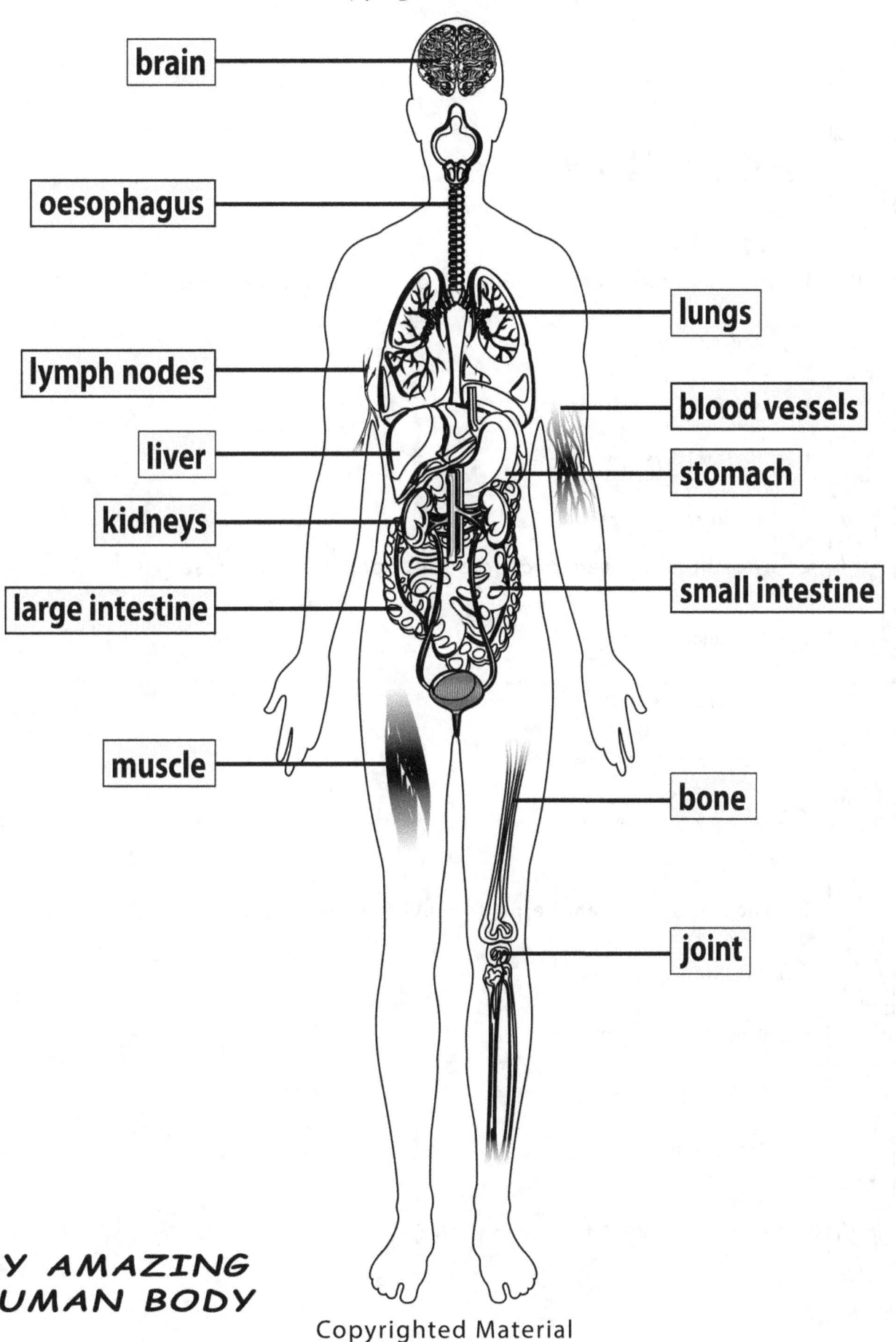

brain

oesophagus

lungs

lymph nodes

blood vessels

liver

stomach

kidneys

large intestine

small intestine

muscle

bone

joint

*MY AMAZING
HUMAN BODY*

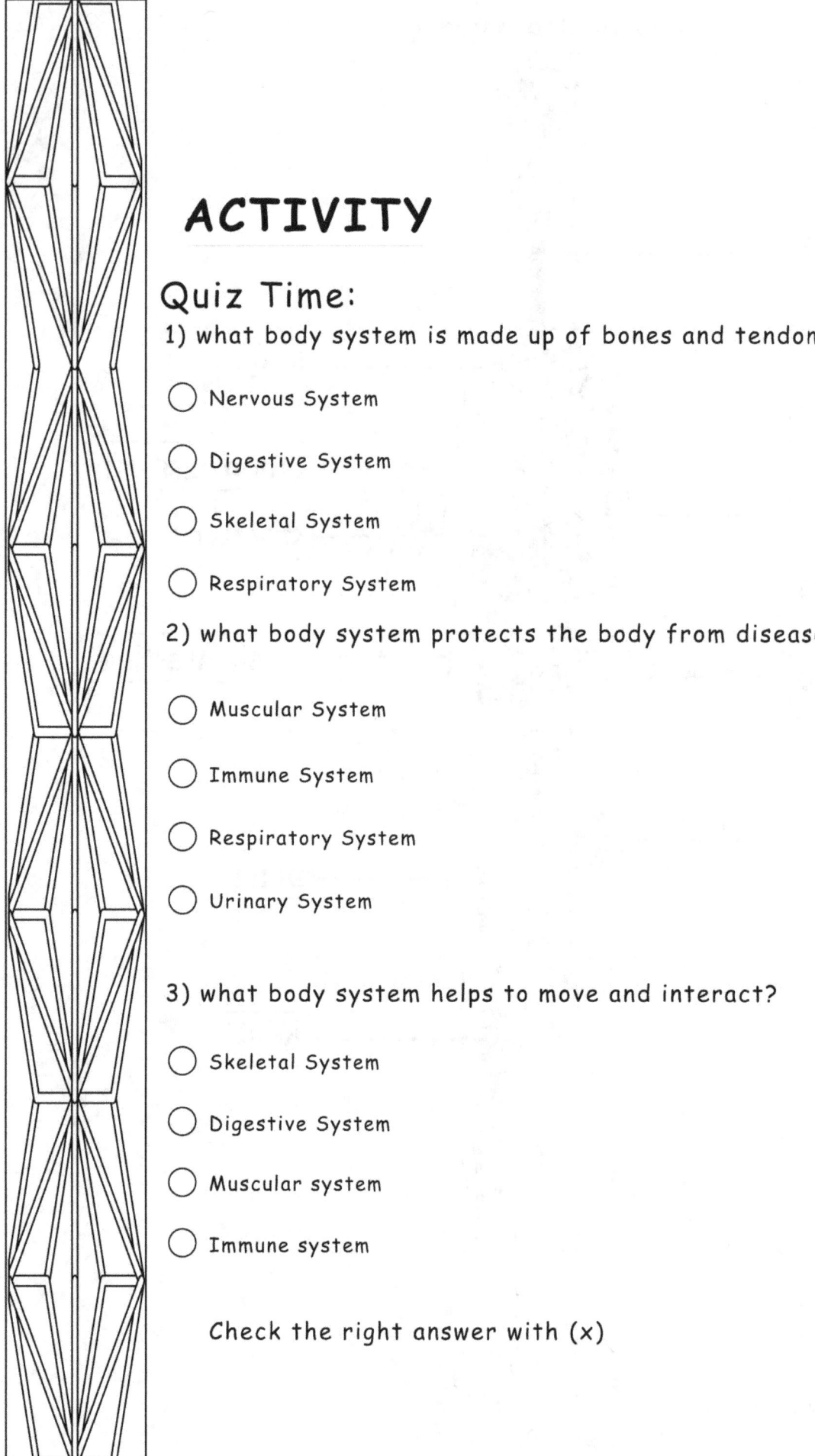

ACTIVITY

Quiz Time:

1) what body system is made up of bones and tendons?

○ Nervous System

○ Digestive System

○ Skeletal System

○ Respiratory System

2) what body system protects the body from disease?

○ Muscular System

○ Immune System

○ Respiratory System

○ Urinary System

3) what body system helps to move and interact?

○ Skeletal System

○ Digestive System

○ Muscular system

○ Immune system

Check the right answer with (x)

Coloring Time

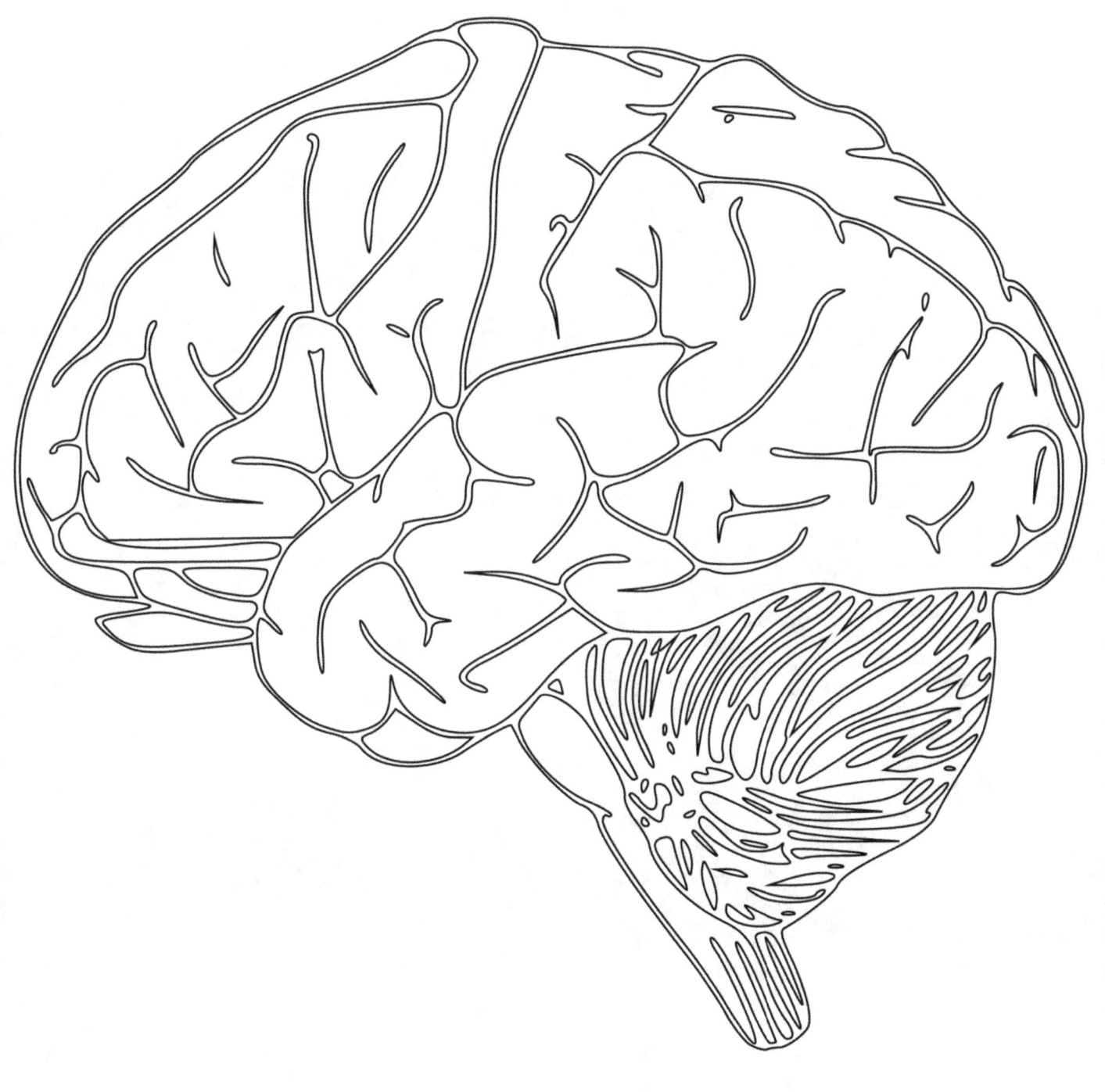

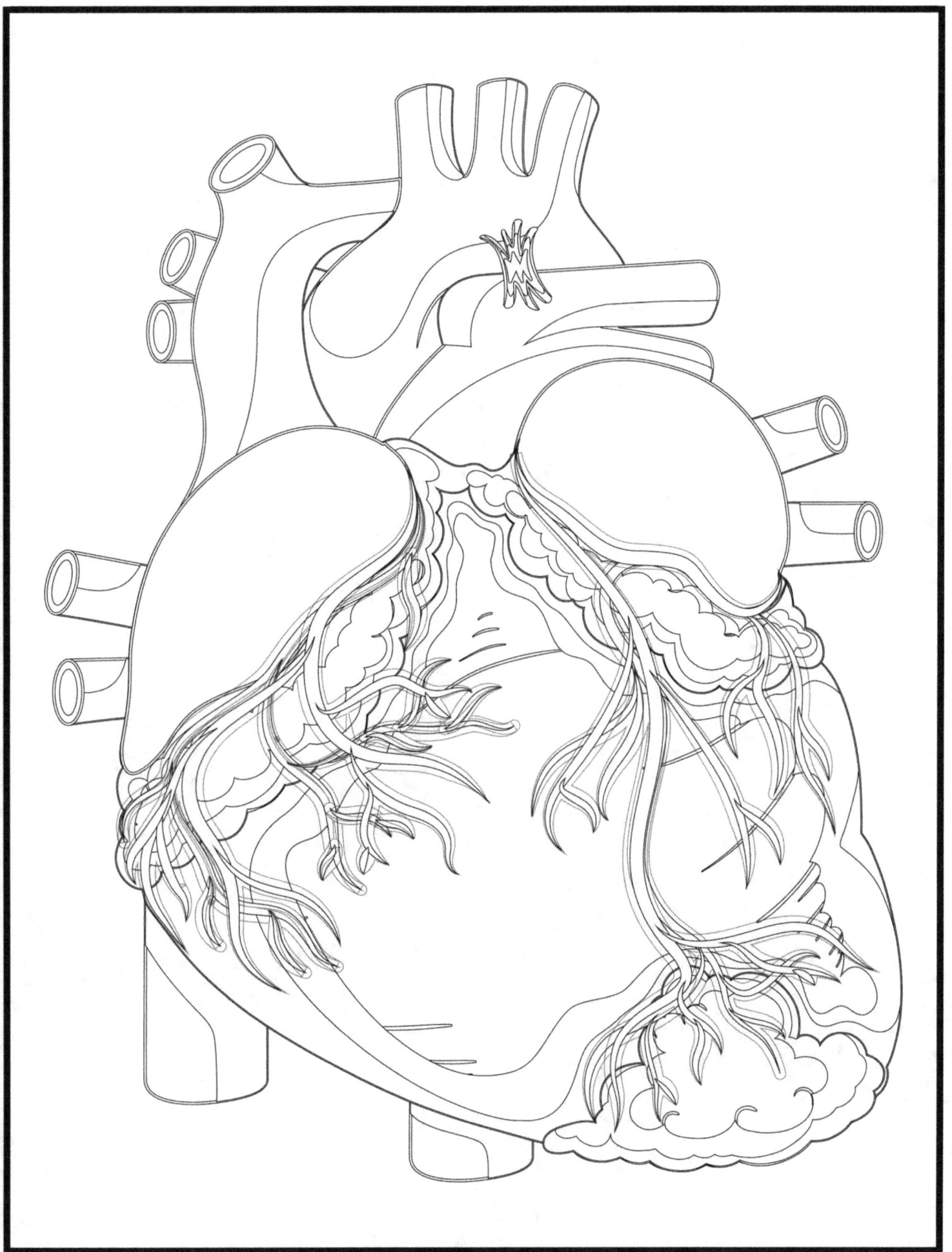

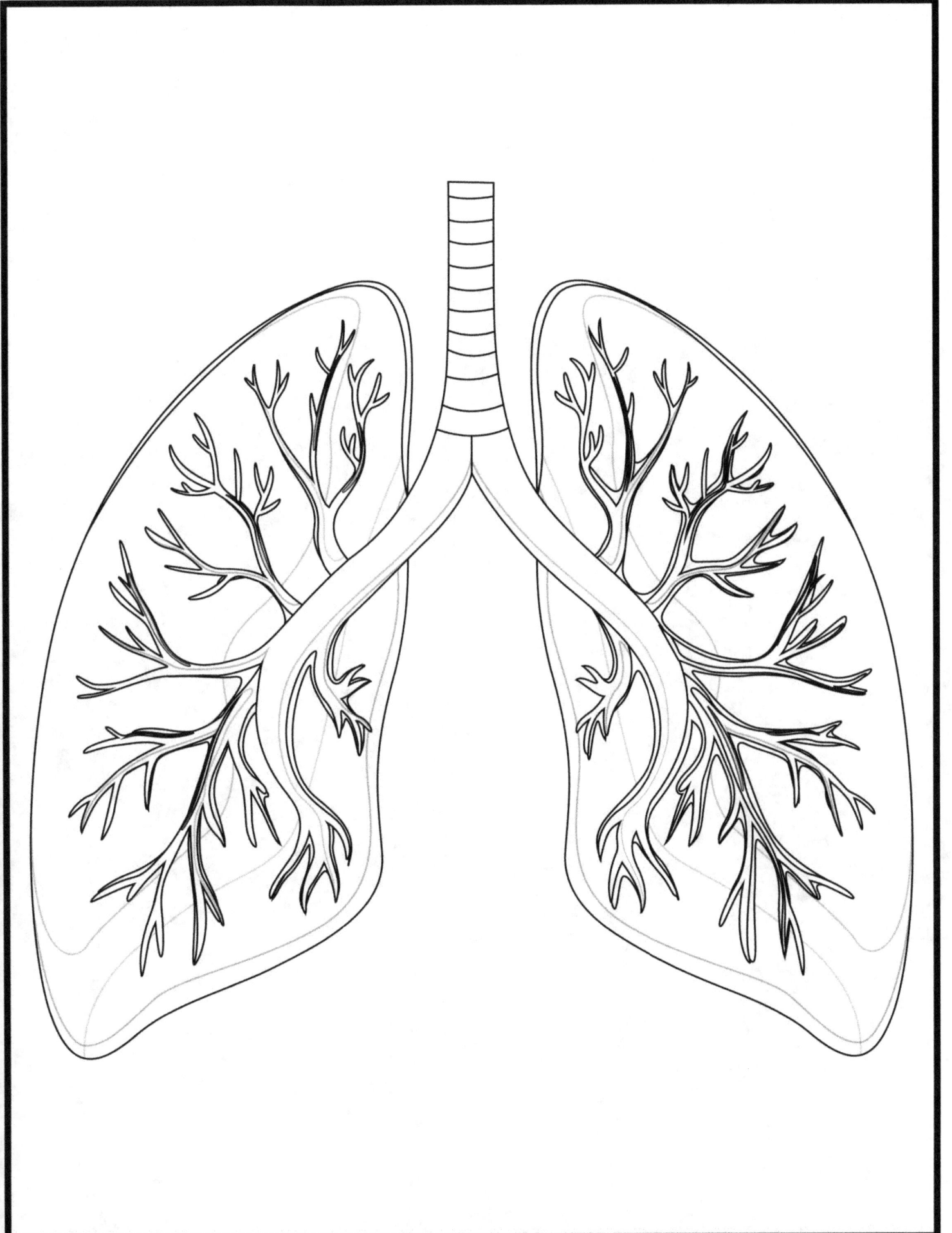

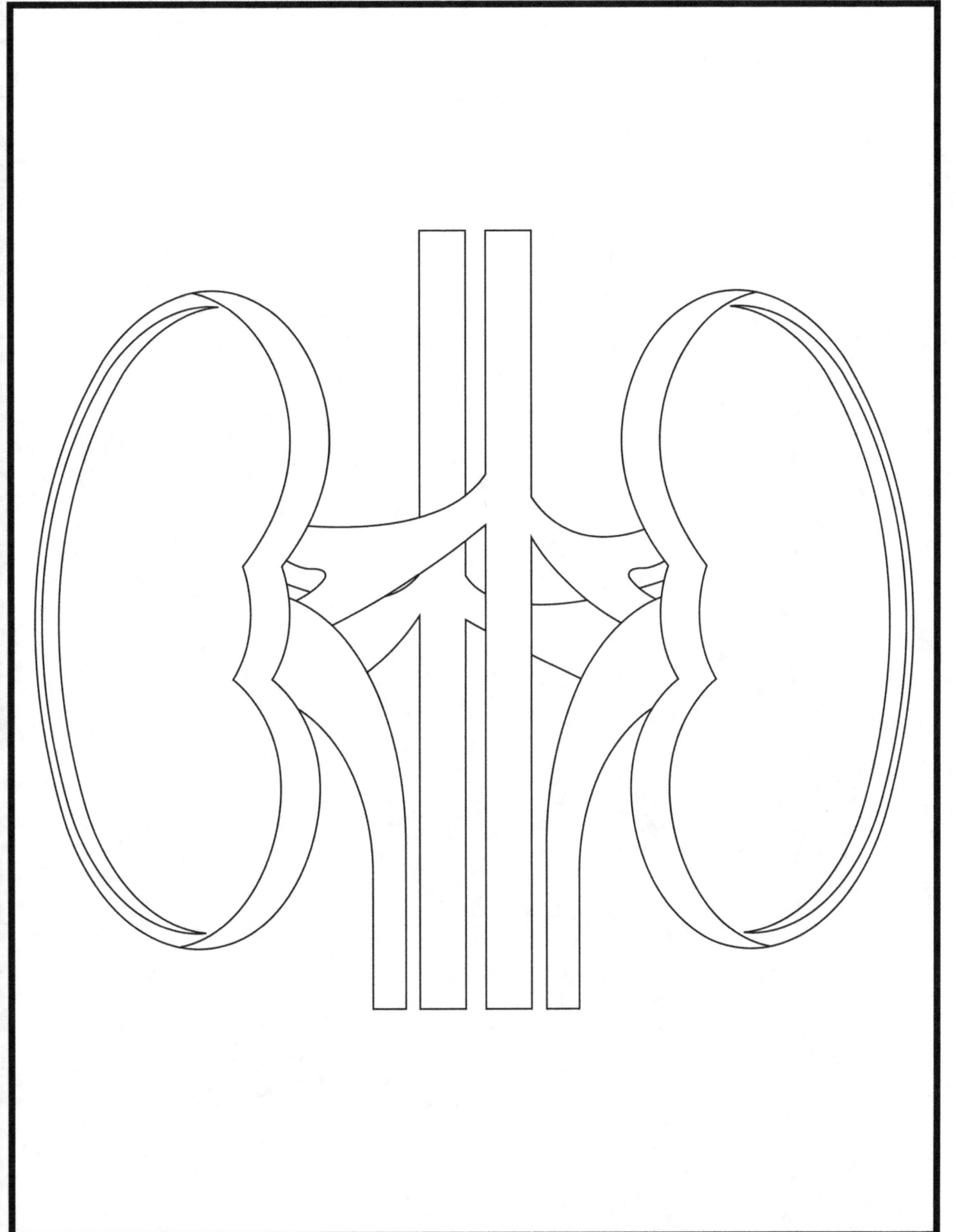

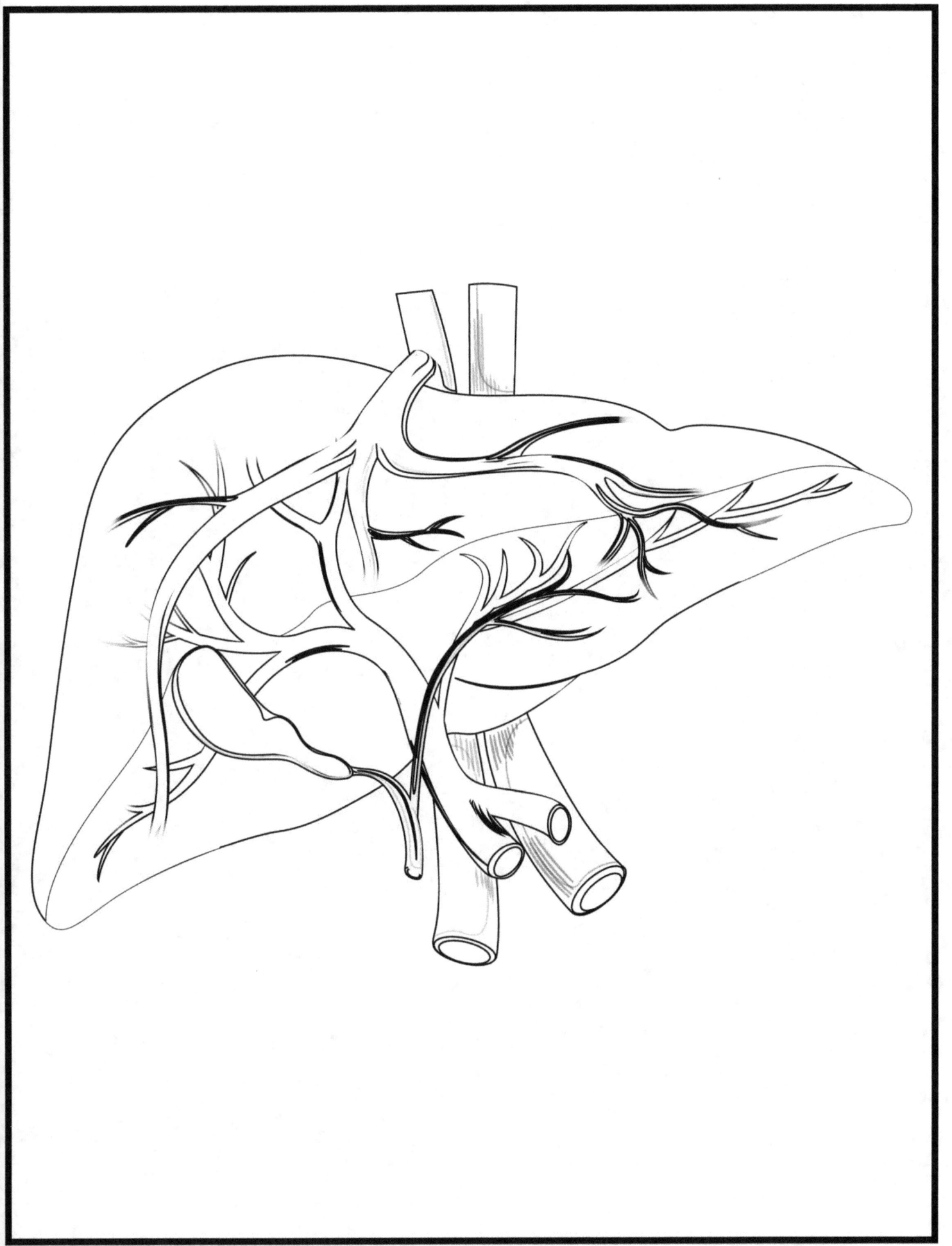

MICROSCOPY CELLS

The cell is the basic unity of life. Some organisms are made up of a single cell, like bacteria, while others are made up of thrillions of cells.

Human beings are made up of cells,too.

Cells provide structure for body, take in nutrients from food and carry out important functions.

Cells group together to form tissues, wich in turn group together to form organs, such as the heart and the brain.

Our cells contain a number of functional structures called organelles.

These organelles carry out tasks such as making proteins, processing chemicals and generating energy for the cell.

Fun Facts

- Every second, your body produces 25 million new cells.

- Cells are the smallest biological unit of life found in all organisms.

- there are two different types of cells eukaryotic or prokaryotic.

- It's estimated the average human body has about 40 trillion cells.

- It's estimated the human brain alone contains 80 billion cells.

Human cells

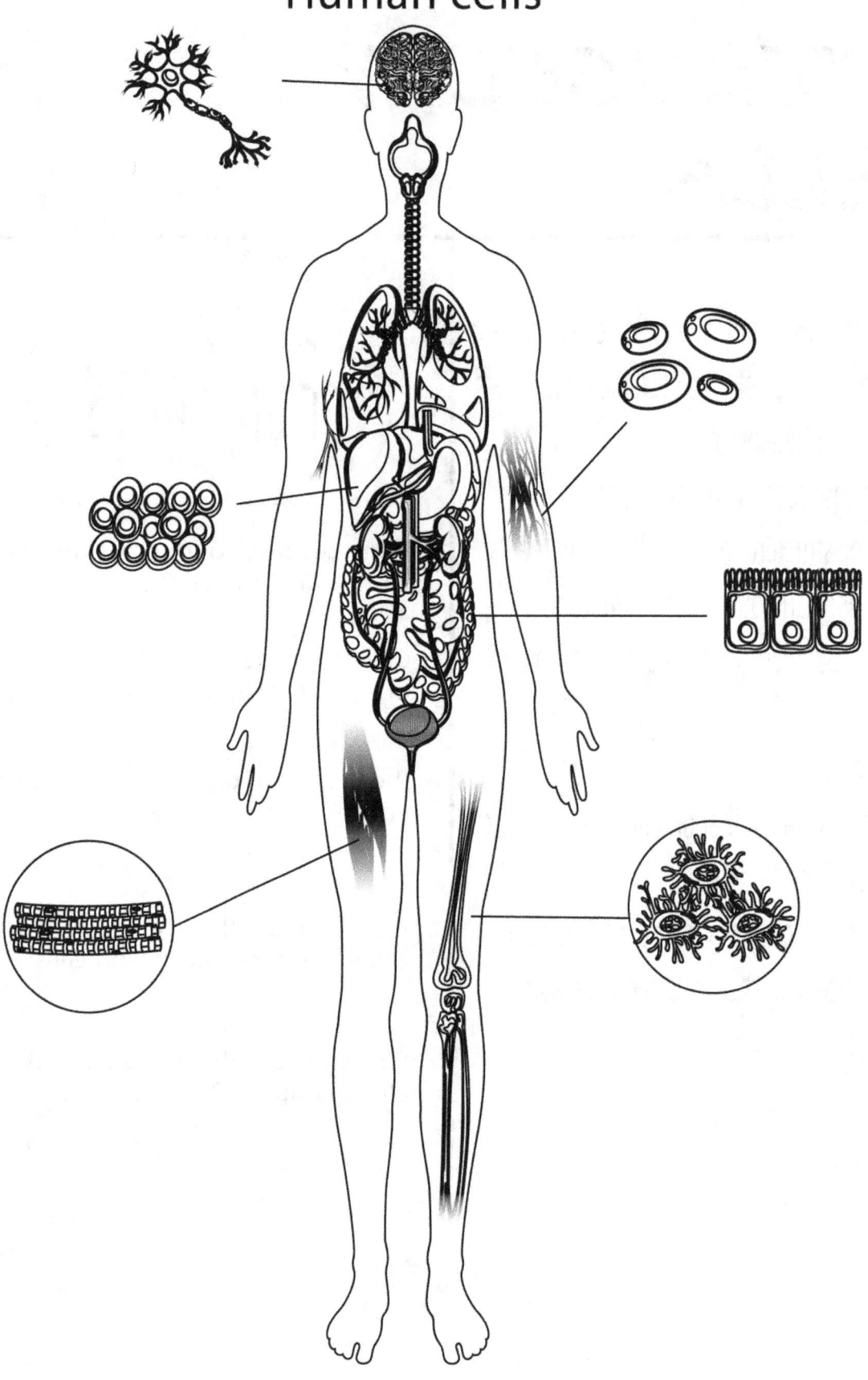

ACTIVITY

*Find these words and complete this word search puzzle

-Nucleus /-Cytoplasm /-Meiosis /-Enzymes /-RNA /-Membrane /-Fission
-Wall /-Cycle /-Division /-Protein /-Cell /-Mitosis /-Diploid /-Organelle
-Flagella /-Chloplast /-Ribosome /-Translation /-Eukatyotic.

O	B	Q	N	C	I	A	Z	L	F	R	L	Y	A	Z	C	P	Q
F	L	Q	P	S	A	M	R	I	B	O	S	O	M	E	W	U	M
S	H	E	R	I	N	E	M	Q	Y	N	N	Q	F	D	O	K	Q
A	J	G	F	S	R	I	E	D	S	O	N	D	J	C	K	M	F
G	K	Z	P	O	W	O	M	N	O	I	S	I	V	I	D	I	D
B	N	K	A	T	W	S	B	B	X	T	G	H	R	H	W	R	S
P	B	O	P	I	L	I	R	C	J	A	L	Z	F	X	R	U	T
A	P	C	I	M	W	S	A	F	H	L	P	R	O	T	E	I	N
Y	F	H	H	S	O	T	N	T	E	S	K	R	T	L	K	B	T
D	M	L	Q	L	S	C	E	C	M	N	C	U	C	J	S	B	K
I	H	M	A	N	O	I	Y	X	J	A	M	U	C	E	W	Q	U
O	X	K	X	G	E	R	F	T	L	R	N	W	M	Y	W	S	T
L	I	V	U	J	E	H	O	M	O	T	A	Y	Q	O	C	H	O
P	V	Z	N	F	W	L	R	P	W	P	Z	V	P	Y	N	L	E
I	A	Q	P	H	C	A	L	V	L	N	L	K	B	C	V	Y	E
D	J	Q	M	K	K	J	L	A	E	A	W	A	P	J	Z	W	O
Q	I	O	R	G	A	N	E	L	L	E	S	K	S	F	J	M	O
A	E	U	K	A	R	Y	O	T	I	C	U	P	T	M	Q	Q	I

ACTIVITY

Quiz Time:

1) which of the following is a function of a nerve cell?

◯ to help us think

◯ to produce enery

◯ to transport messages around the body

◯ to help us move

2) the nucleus is to the cell as the _____ to the body.

◯ lungs

◯ eyes

◯ brain

◯ stomach

3) which of the following is not made up of eukaryotic cells ?

◯ animals

◯ bacteria

◯ plants

◯ non of the above

Check the right answer with (x)

Coloring Time

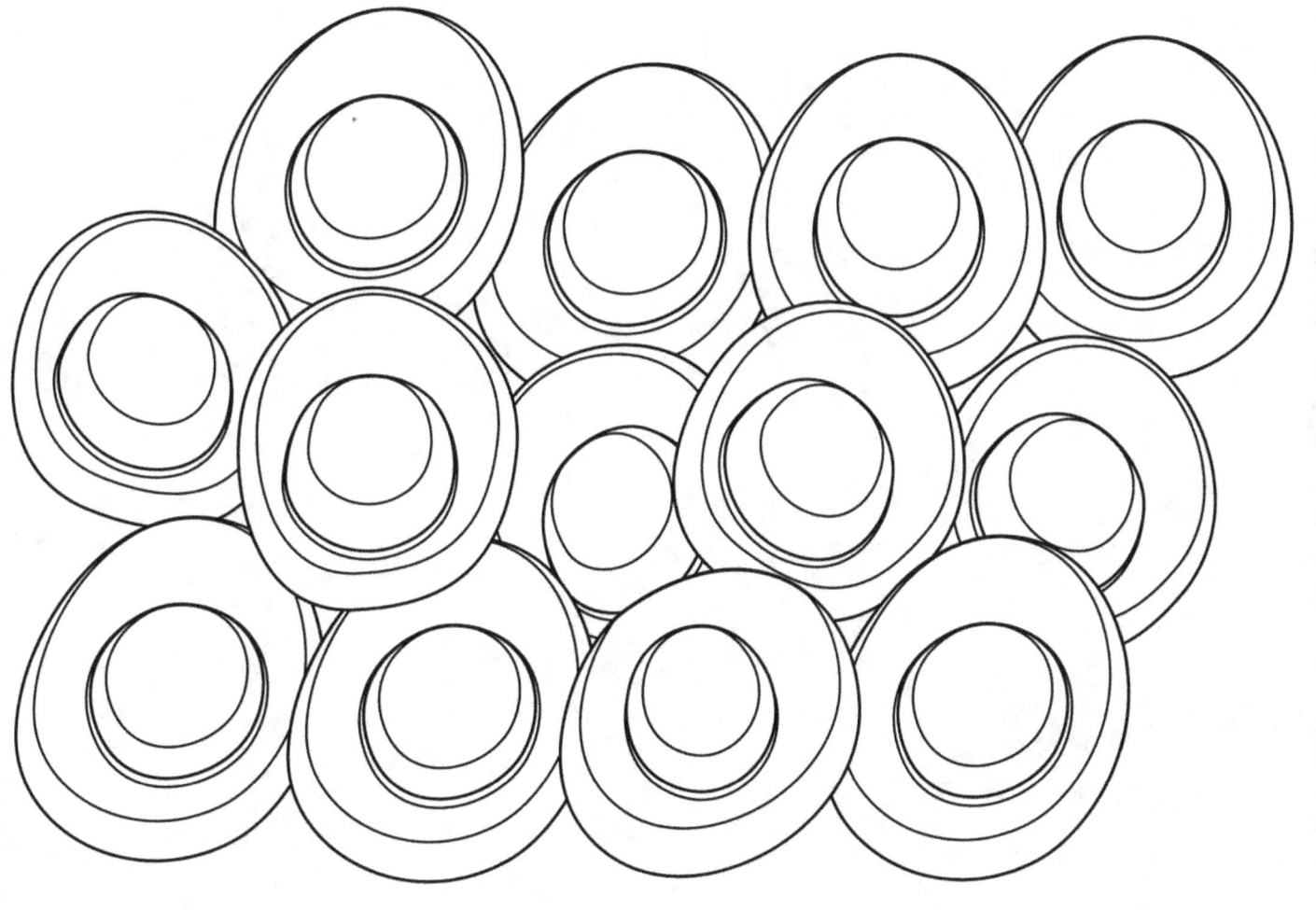

Liver Cells

Coloring Time

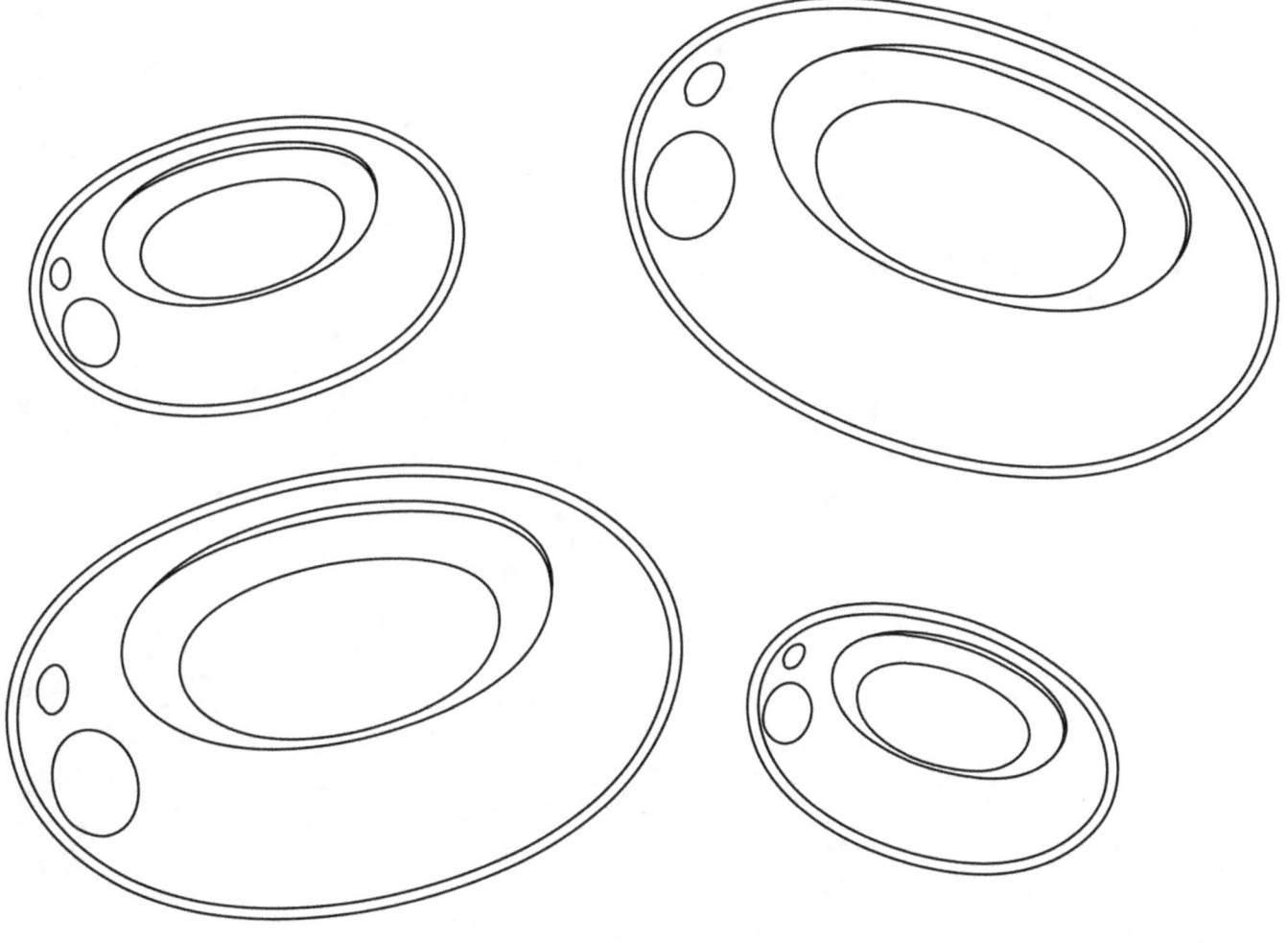

Blood Cells

Coloring Time

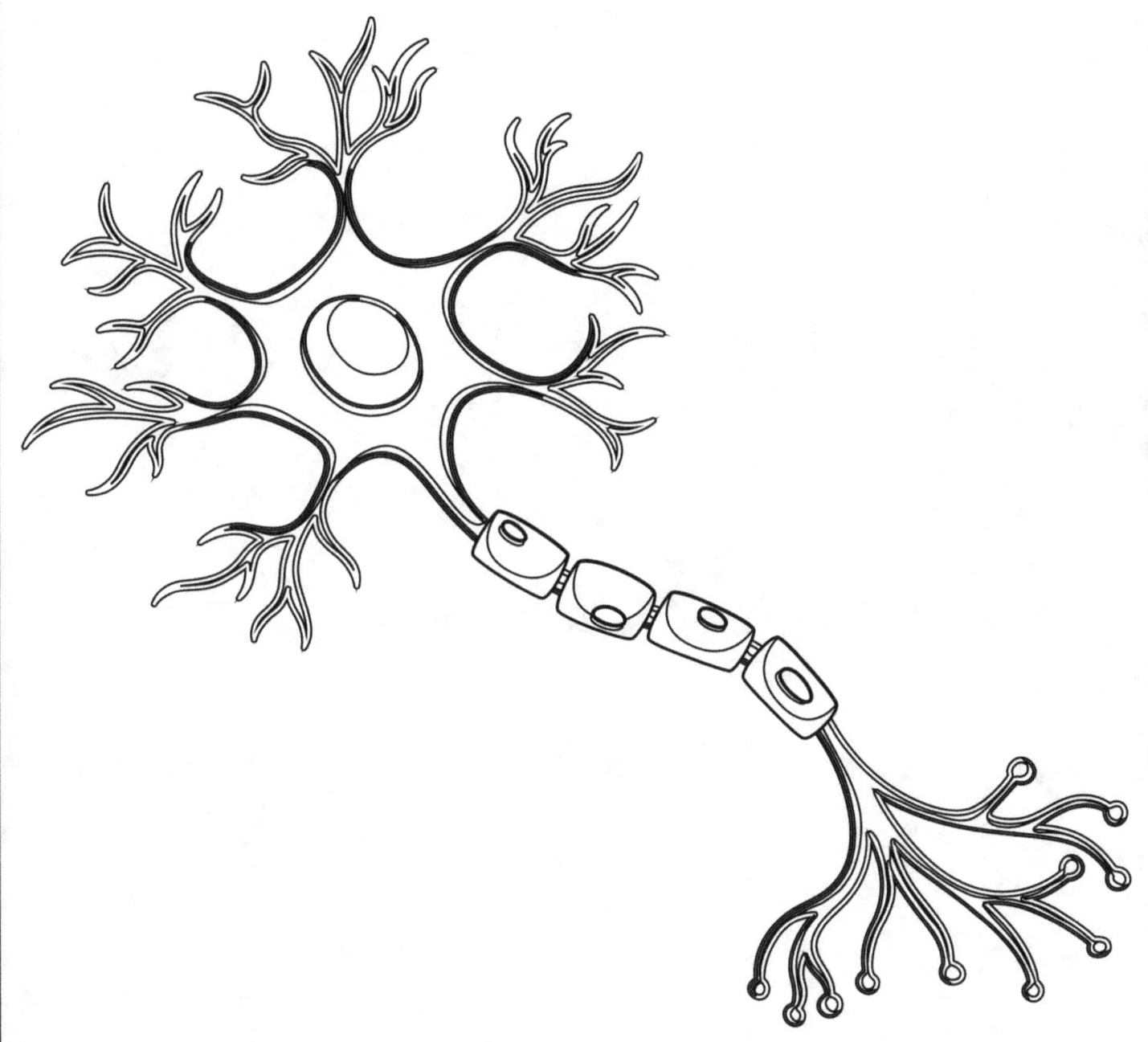

Brain Cells

MY FOUNDATION
OUR SKELETON

The human skeleton is the internal framework of the human body. It is composed of around 300 bones at birth this total decreases to around 206 bones by adulthood after some bones get fused together. The bone mass in the skeleton reaches maximum density around age 21. The human skeleton can be divided into the axial skeleton and the appendicular skeleton. around 70 percent of your bones are not living tissue, but har minerals like calcium. The outside of the bones is called the cortical bone. It's hard, smooth and solid. Inside the cortical bone is a porous, spongy bone material called the trabecular or concellous bone.

Fun Facts

- ✦ The smallest bone found in the human body is located in the middle ear.

- ✦ The femur is the longest bone in the human body.

- ✦ More than half of your bones are located in the hands,writs,feet,ankles

- ✦ Infants are born with approximately 300 bones but as they grow some of these bones fuse together.

- ✦ Joints are the place where two bones meets or connect.

Human skeletal system

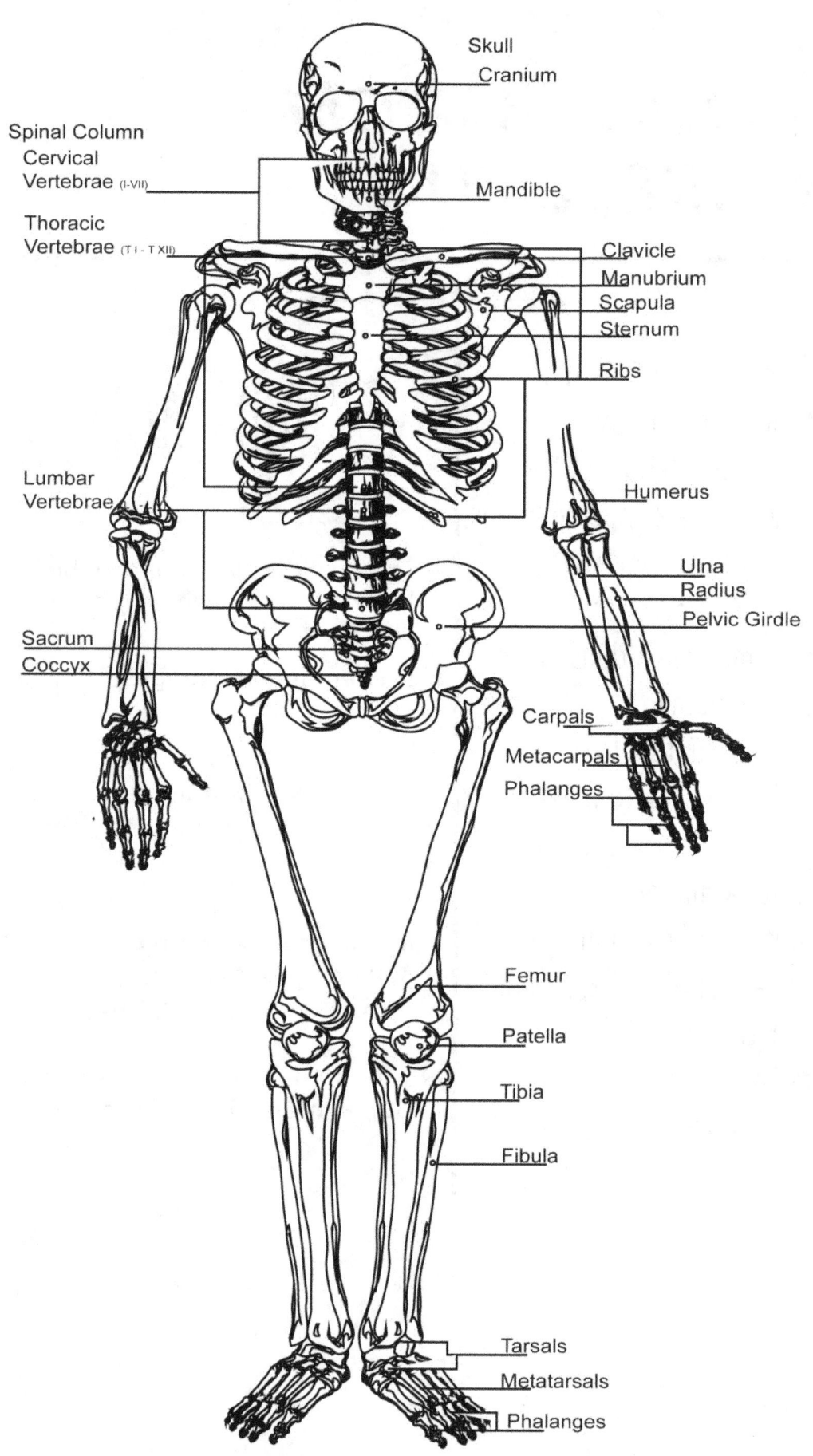

Skull
Cranium

Spinal Column
Cervical
Vertebrae (I-VII)

Mandible

Thoracic
Vertebrae (T I - T XII)

Clavicle
Manubrium
Scapula
Sternum

Ribs

Lumbar
Vertebrae

Humerus

Ulna
Radius
Pelvic Girdle

Sacrum
Coccyx

Carpals

Metacarpals

Phalanges

Femur

Patella

Tibia

Fibula

Tarsals

Metatarsals

Phalanges

Human skeletal system

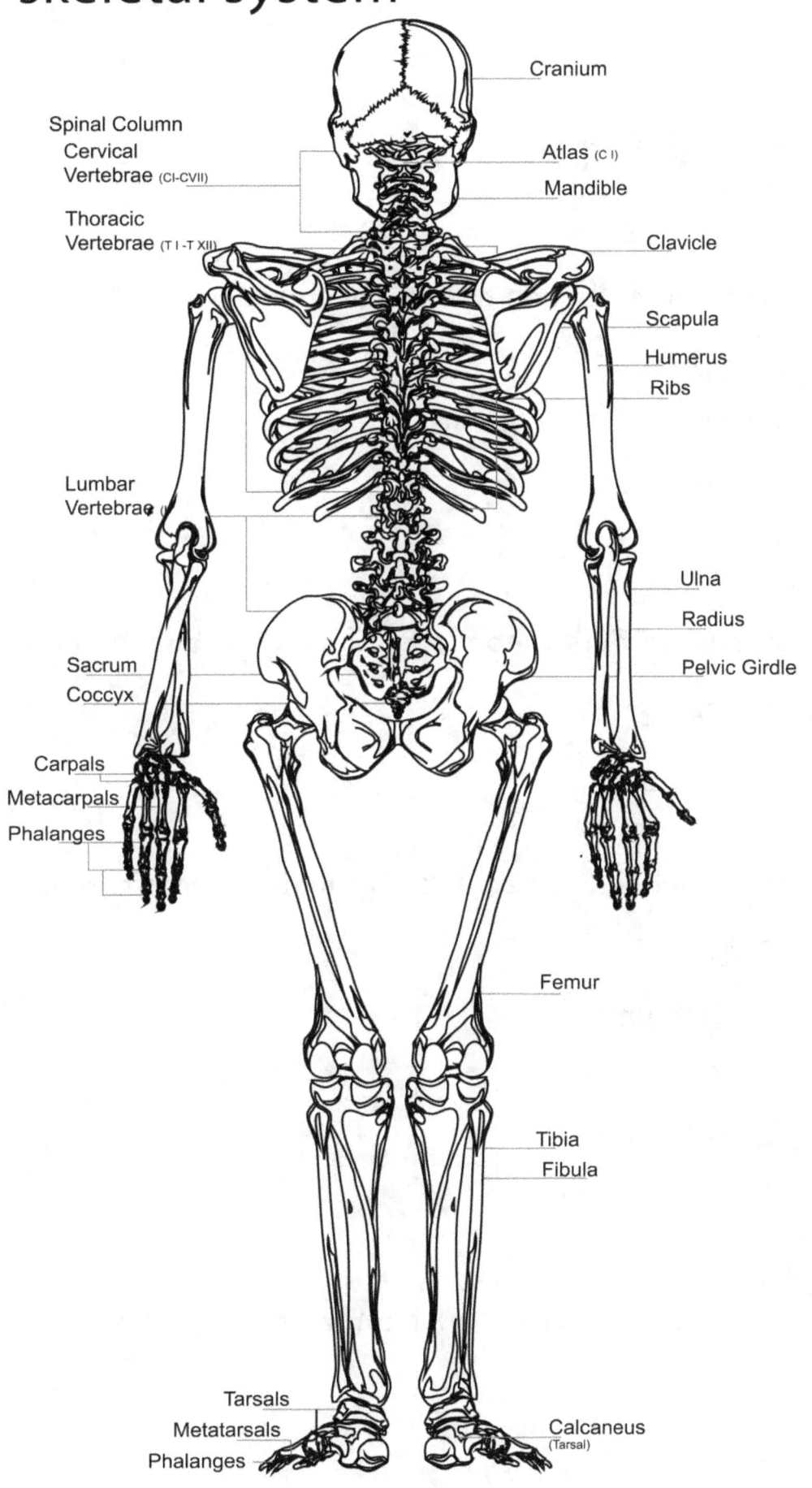

Cranium

Spinal Column
Cervical
Vertebrae (CI-CVII)

Atlas (C I)

Mandible

Thoracic
Vertebrae (T I -T XII)

Clavicle

Scapula

Humerus

Ribs

Lumbar
Vertebrae

Ulna

Radius

Pelvic Girdle

Sacrum

Coccyx

Carpals

Metacarpals

Phalanges

Femur

Tibia

Fibula

Tarsals

Metatarsals

Phalanges

Calcaneus
(Tarsal)

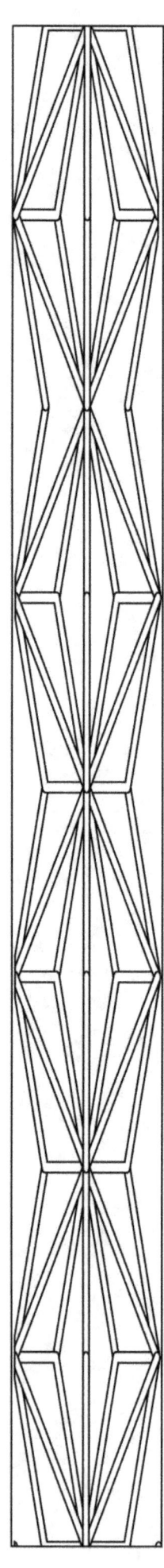

ACTIVITY

Quiz Time:

1) How many bones are in the human body ?

○ 115

○ 45

○ 206

○ 500

2)True or False: about 85% of your bones are living tessue.

○ TRUE

○ FALSE

3) what hard mineral is the main element in our bones?

○ Iron

○ Calcium

○ Zinc

○ Potassium

Check the right answer with (x)

Name and Color the bones

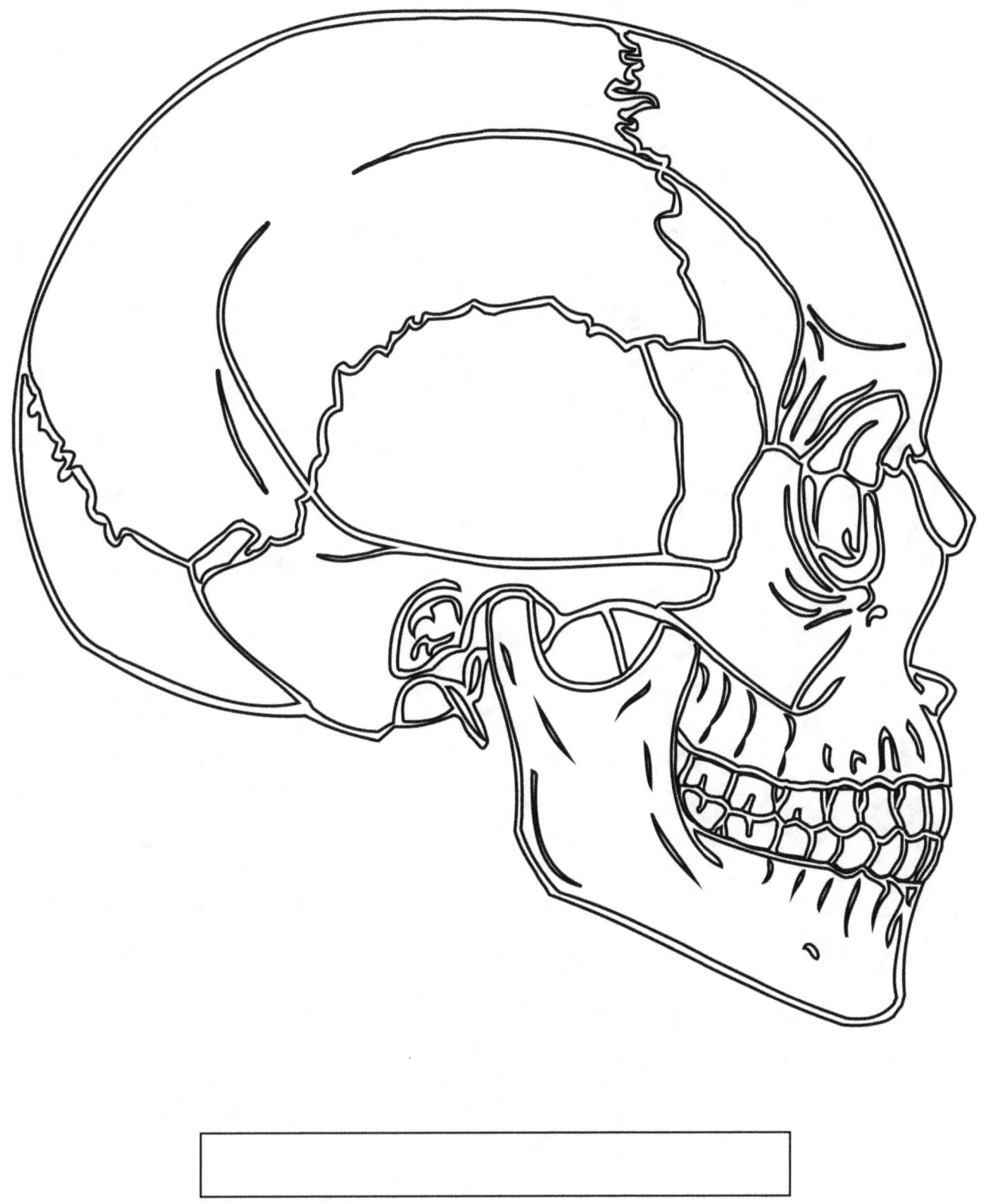

Name and Color the bones

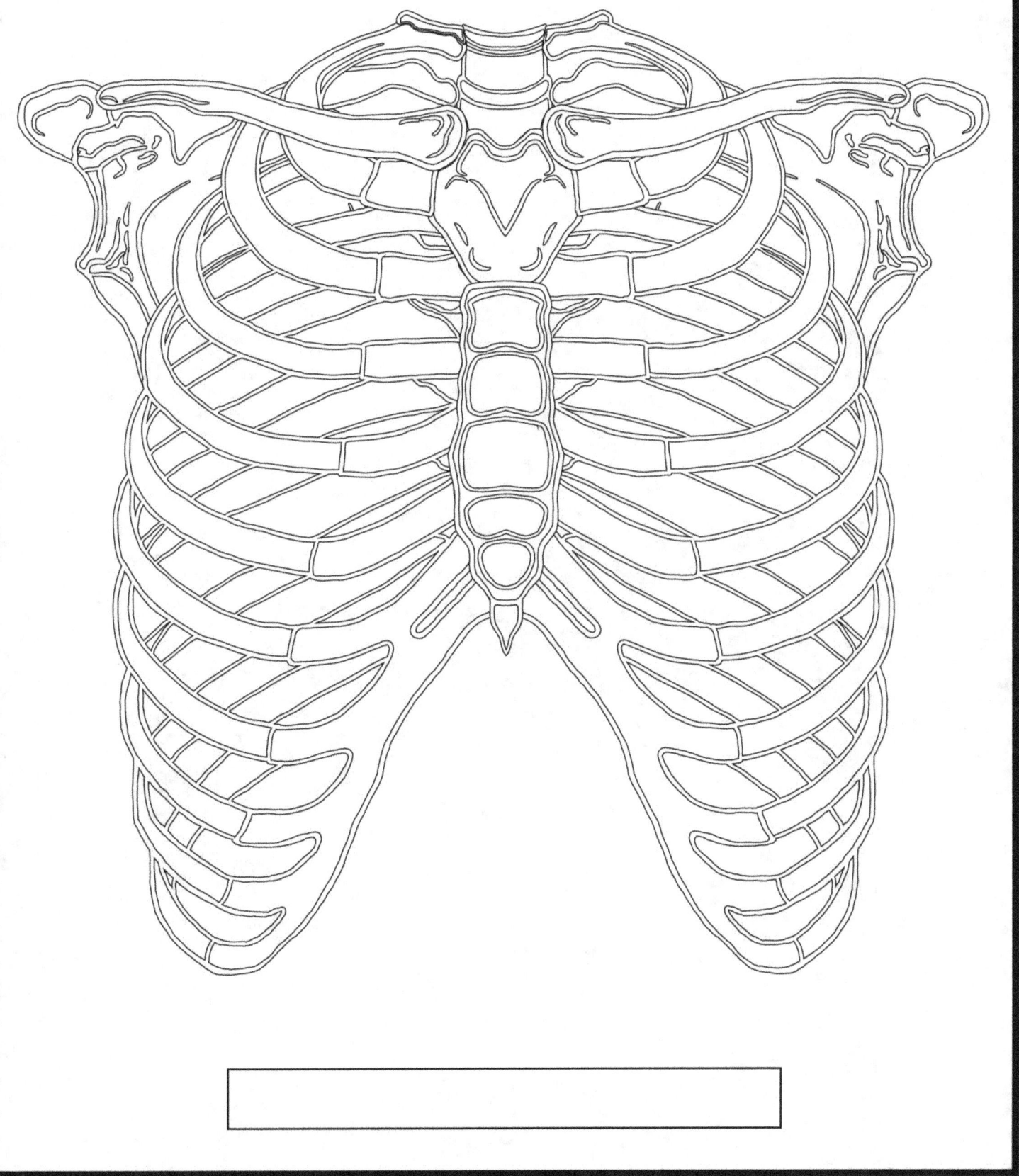

Name and Color the bones

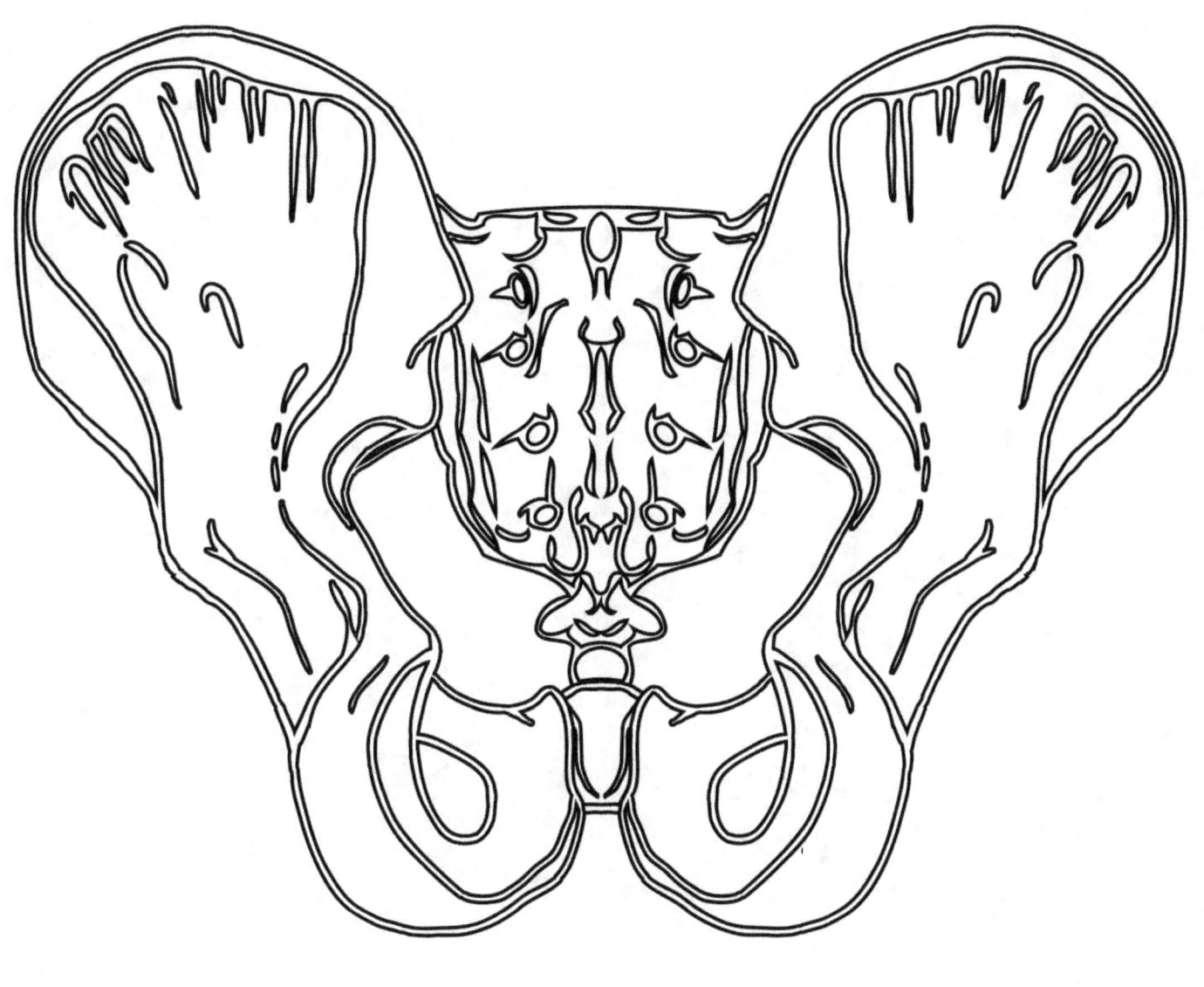

OUR STRONG MUSCLES

Muscles are how we move and live. All movement in the body is controlled be muscles some muscles work without us thinking, like our heart beating, while other muscles are controlled by our thoughts and allow us to do stuff and move around all of our muscles tohether make up the body's muscular system. There are over 650 muscles in the human body. They are under our skin and cover our bones. Muscles often work together to help us move. We can't really have to think about moving each indivivual muscle. For example, we just think of running and our body does the rest. The muscular system is an organ system consisting of skeletal, smooth and cardiac muscles. It permits movment of the body, maintains posture and circulates blood throughout the body. The muscular systems in vertebrates are controlled through the nervous system although some muscles such as the cardiac muscle can be completly autonomous. Together with the skeletal system it forms the musculoskeletal system, which is responsibale fo movement of the human body.

Fun Facts

◆ Muscles are divided into three types: smooth, cardiac, and skeletal

◆ Muscles are made up of special cells called muscle fibers

◆ The largest muscle in the body is the gluteus maximus

◆ Muscles are attached to bones by tendons

◆ The hardest working muscle in the body is the heart

Muscular System

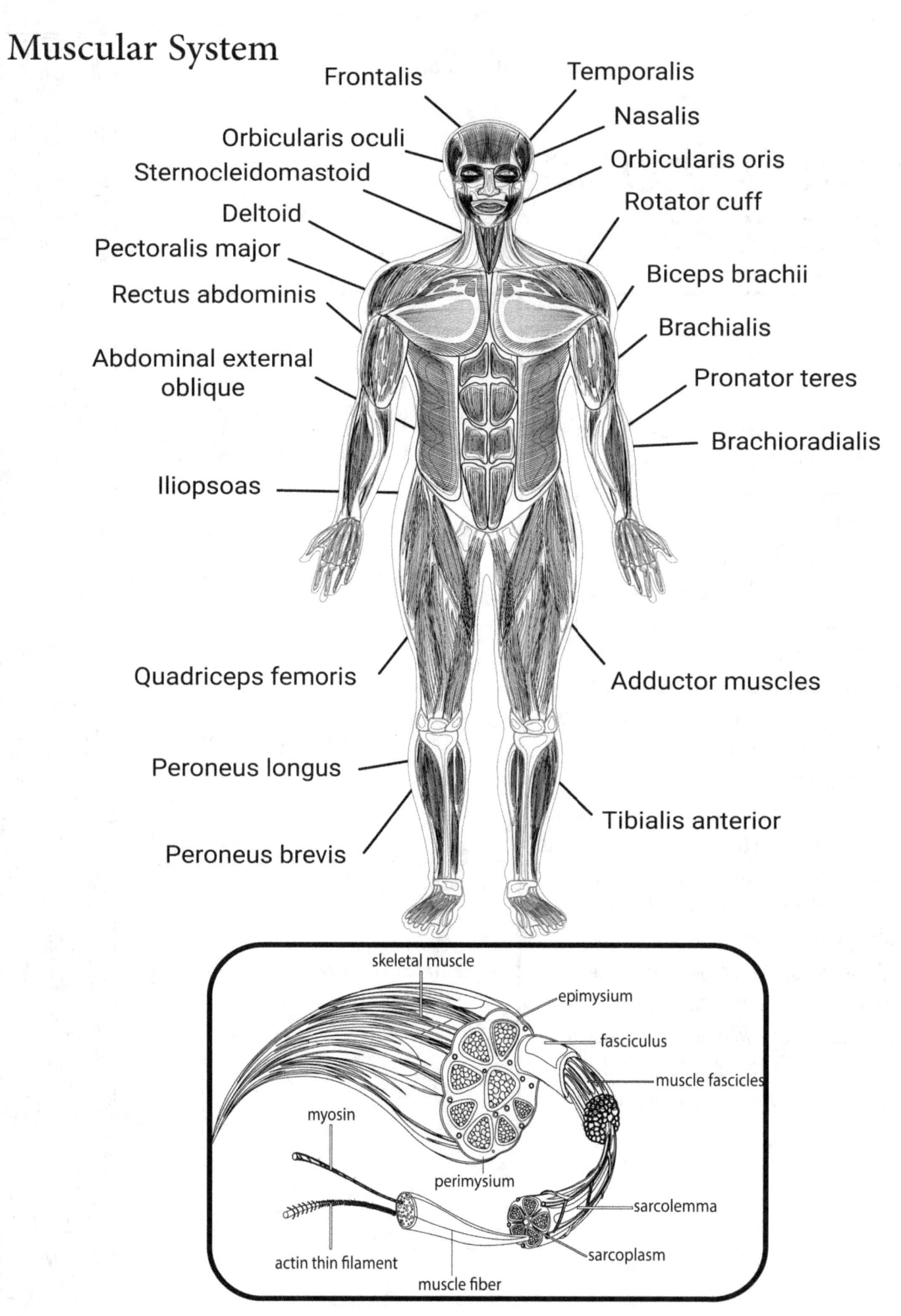

Frontalis

Temporalis

Nasalis

Orbicularis oculi

Orbicularis oris

Sternocleidomastoid

Rotator cuff

Deltoid

Pectoralis major

Biceps brachii

Rectus abdominis

Brachialis

Abdominal external oblique

Pronator teres

Brachioradialis

Iliopsoas

Quadriceps femoris

Adductor muscles

Peroneus longus

Tibialis anterior

Peroneus brevis

skeletal muscle

epimysium

fasciculus

muscle fascicles

myosin

perimysium

sarcolemma

actin thin filament

sarcoplasm

muscle fiber

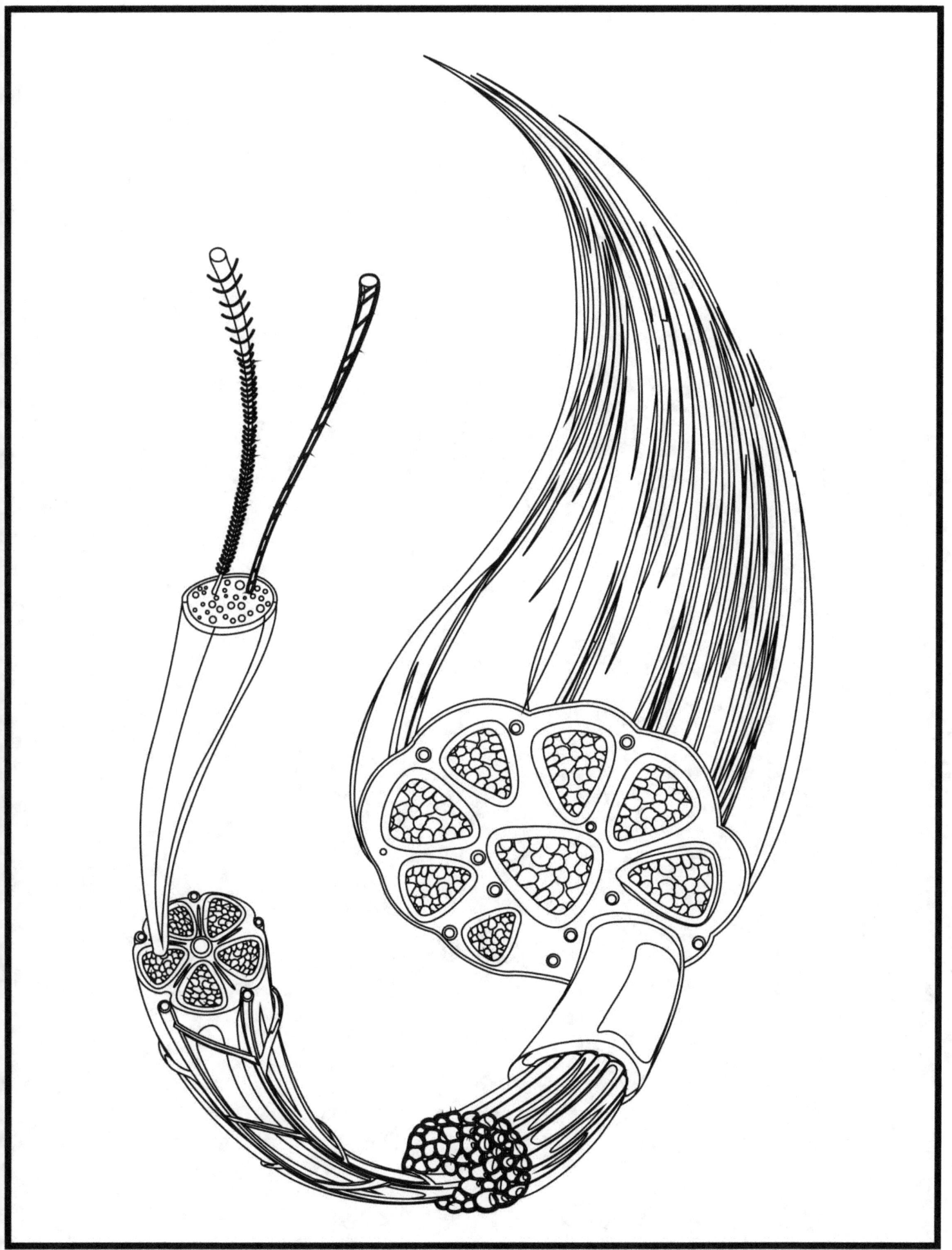

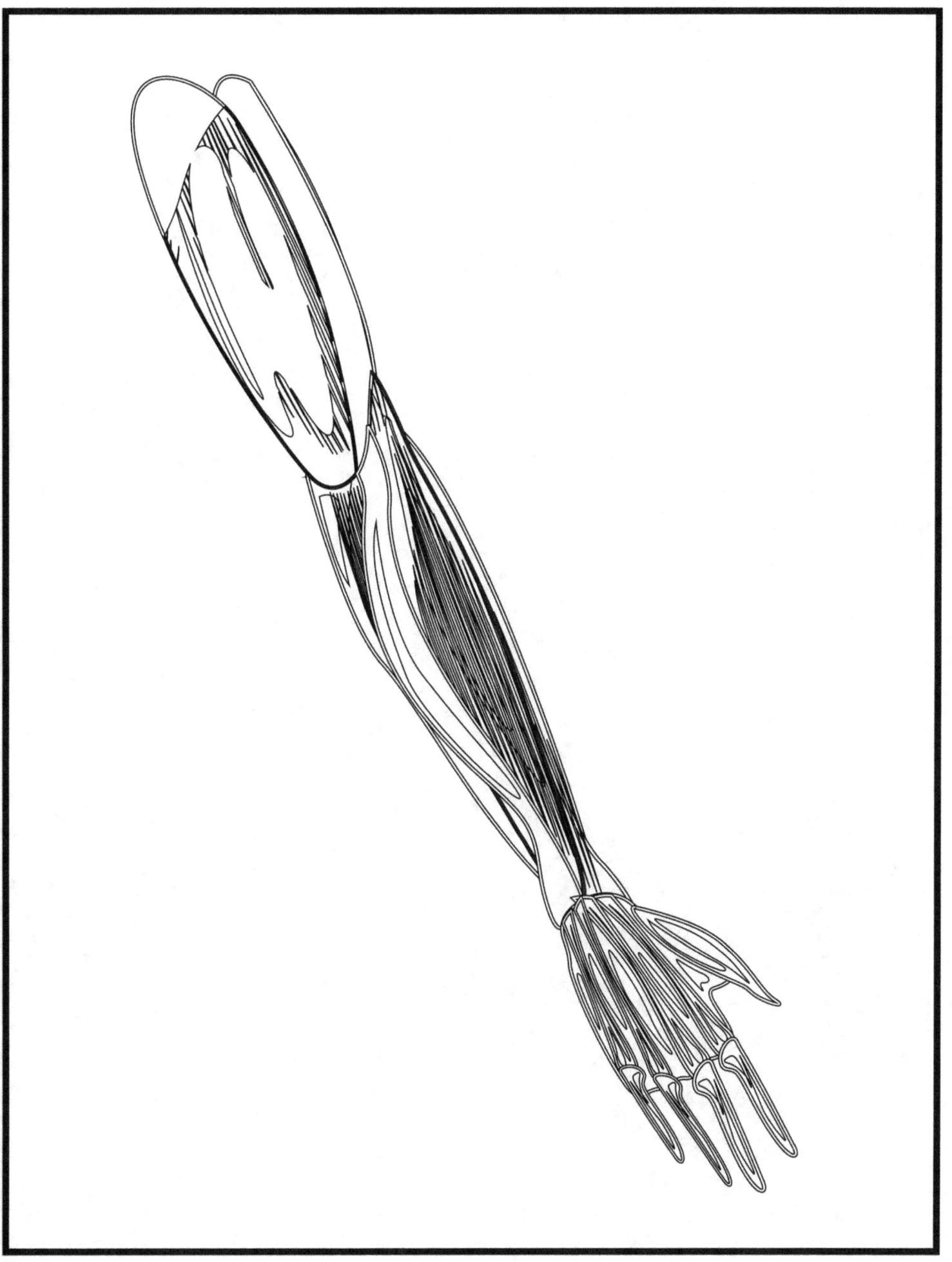

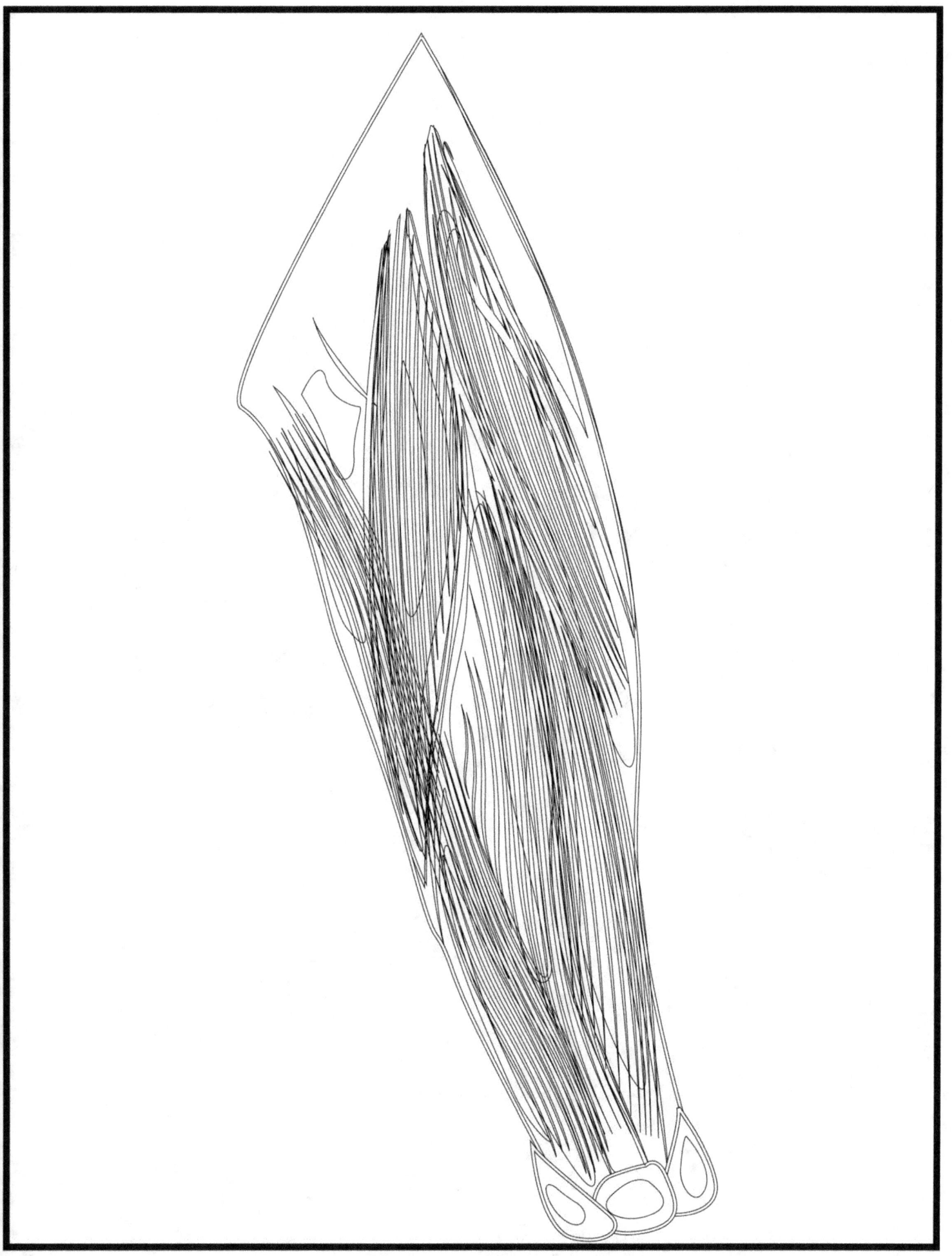

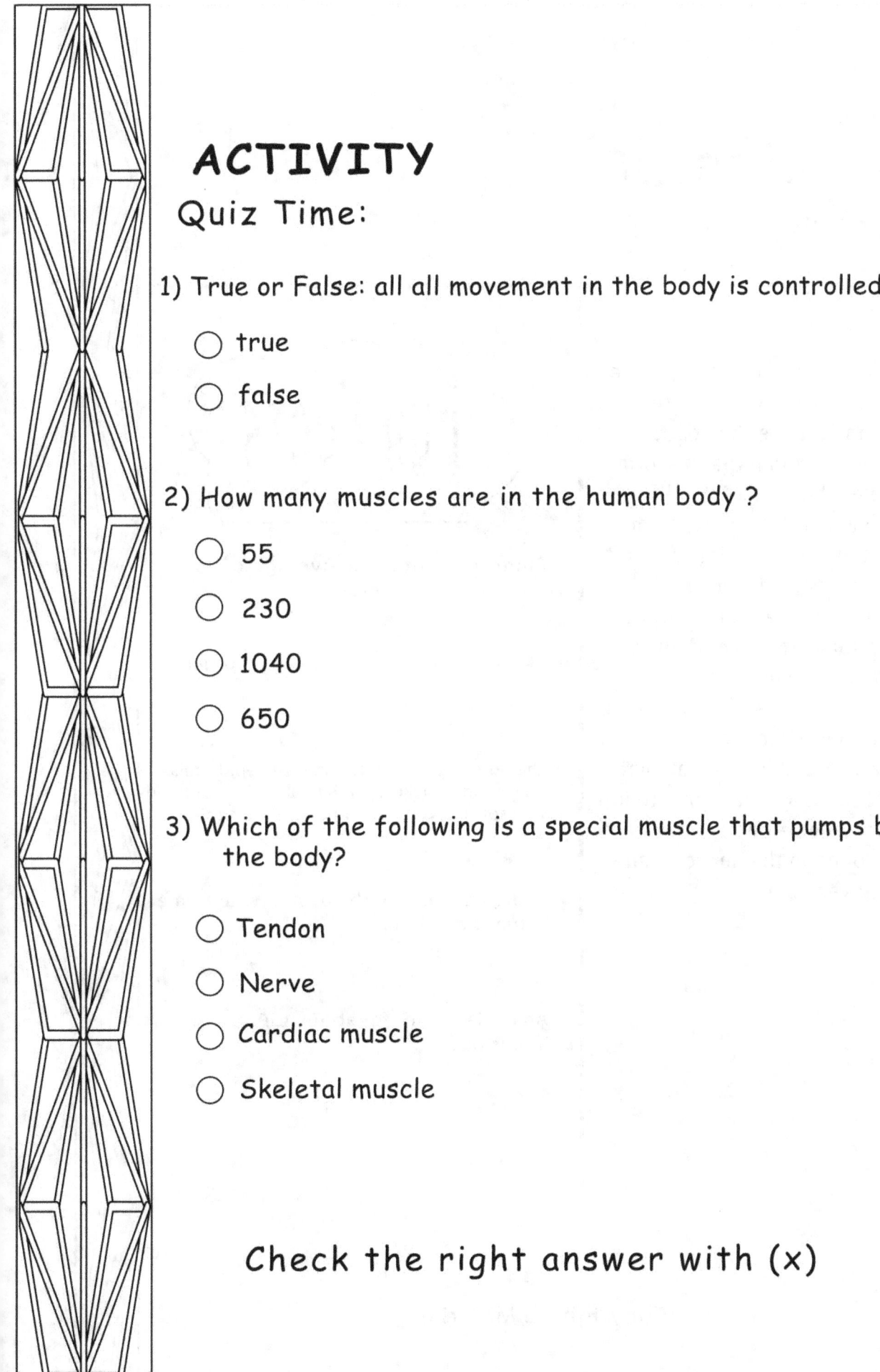

ACTIVITY

Quiz Time:

1) True or False: all all movement in the body is controlled by muscles

    ○ true

    ○ false

2) How many muscles are in the human body ?

    ○ 55

    ○ 230

    ○ 1040

    ○ 650

3) Which of the following is a special muscle that pumps blood through the body?

    ○ Tendon

    ○ Nerve

    ○ Cardiac muscle

    ○ Skeletal muscle

Check the right answer with (x)

HUMAN OUTSIDES
(Hair, nails, skin)

We all have skin. It covers our entire body and keeps the good stuff in and the bad stuff out. The skin is an organ.Just like the heart or the brain. It's an important organ that performs many finctions to enable us to live.
Hair is a protein filament that grows from follicles found in the dermis. Hair is one of the defining characteristics of mammals. The human body, apart from areas of glabrous skin, is covered in follicles which produce thick terminal and fine vellus hair.
A nail is a claw-like kratinous plate at the tip of the fingers and toes in most primates. Nails correspond to claws found in other animals. Fingernails and toenails are made of a tough protective protein called alpha-keratin which is a polymer and found in the hooves, hair, claws and horns of vertebrates.

Fun Facts

◆ Fingernails grow an average o 3.5 millimeters per month.

◆ Skin is the human body's largest organ.

◆ the outer layer of your skin is the epidermis, its is found thickest on the palms of your hands and soles of your feet around 1.5mm thick.

◆ A large amount of the dust in your home is actually dead skin.

◆ An eyelash lives for about 150 days before it falls out .

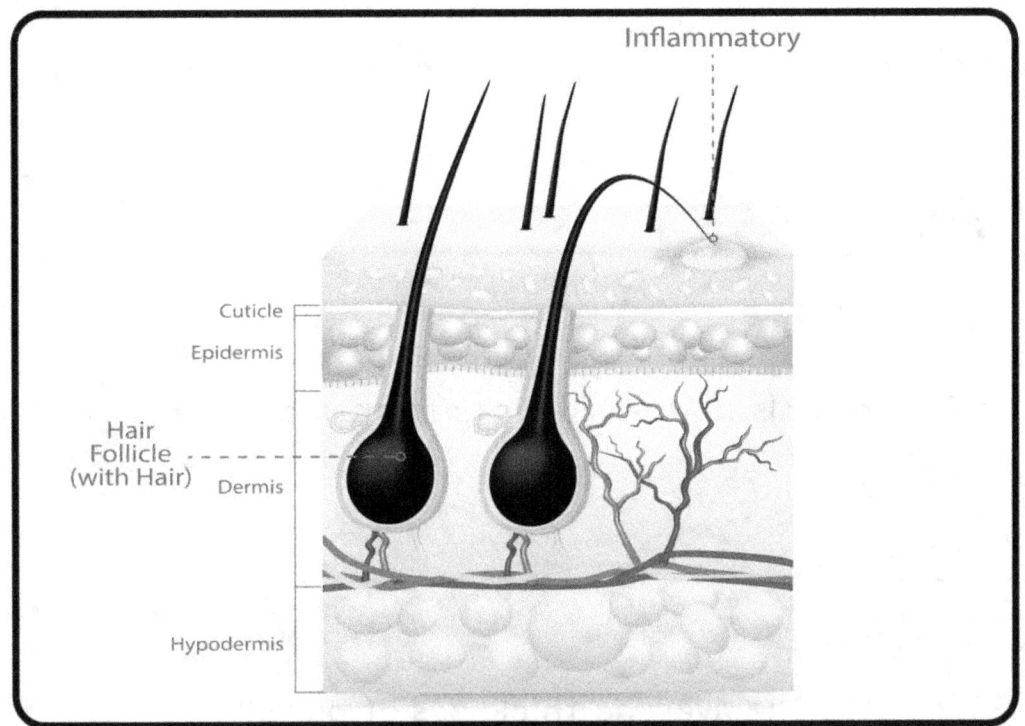

Inflammatory

Cuticle

Epidermis

Hair
Follicle
(with Hair)

Dermis

Hypodermis

Structure of the Hair

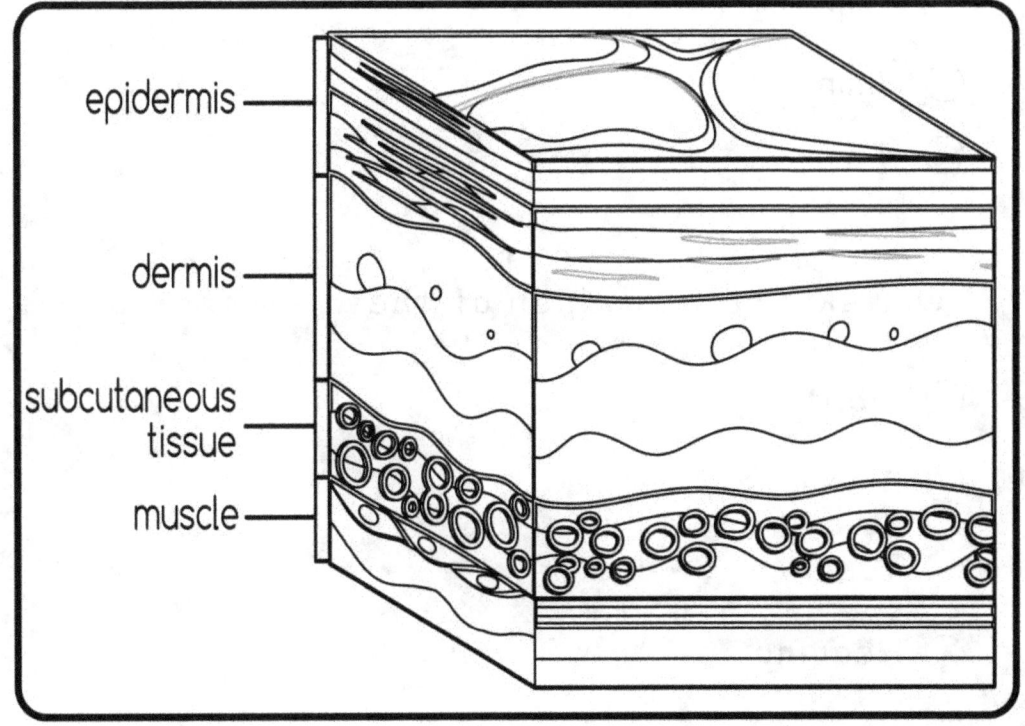

epidermis

dermis

subcutaneous
tissue

muscle

Layers of the human skin

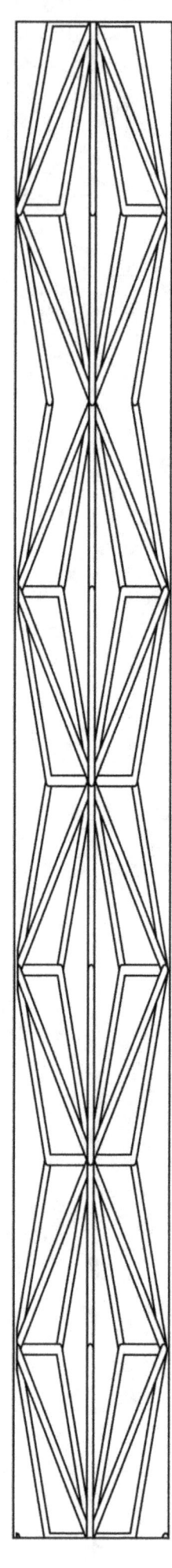

ACTIVITY

Quiz Time:

1) True or False : the skin is not considered an organ like the heart

   ○ True

   ○ False

2) What is the average thickness of our skin

   ○ 1 mm

   ○ 2mm

   ○ 3mm

   ○ 4 mm

3) Our skin houses which of these senses?

   ○ Sight

   ○ Smell

   ○ Touch

   ○ Hearing

Check the right answer with (x)

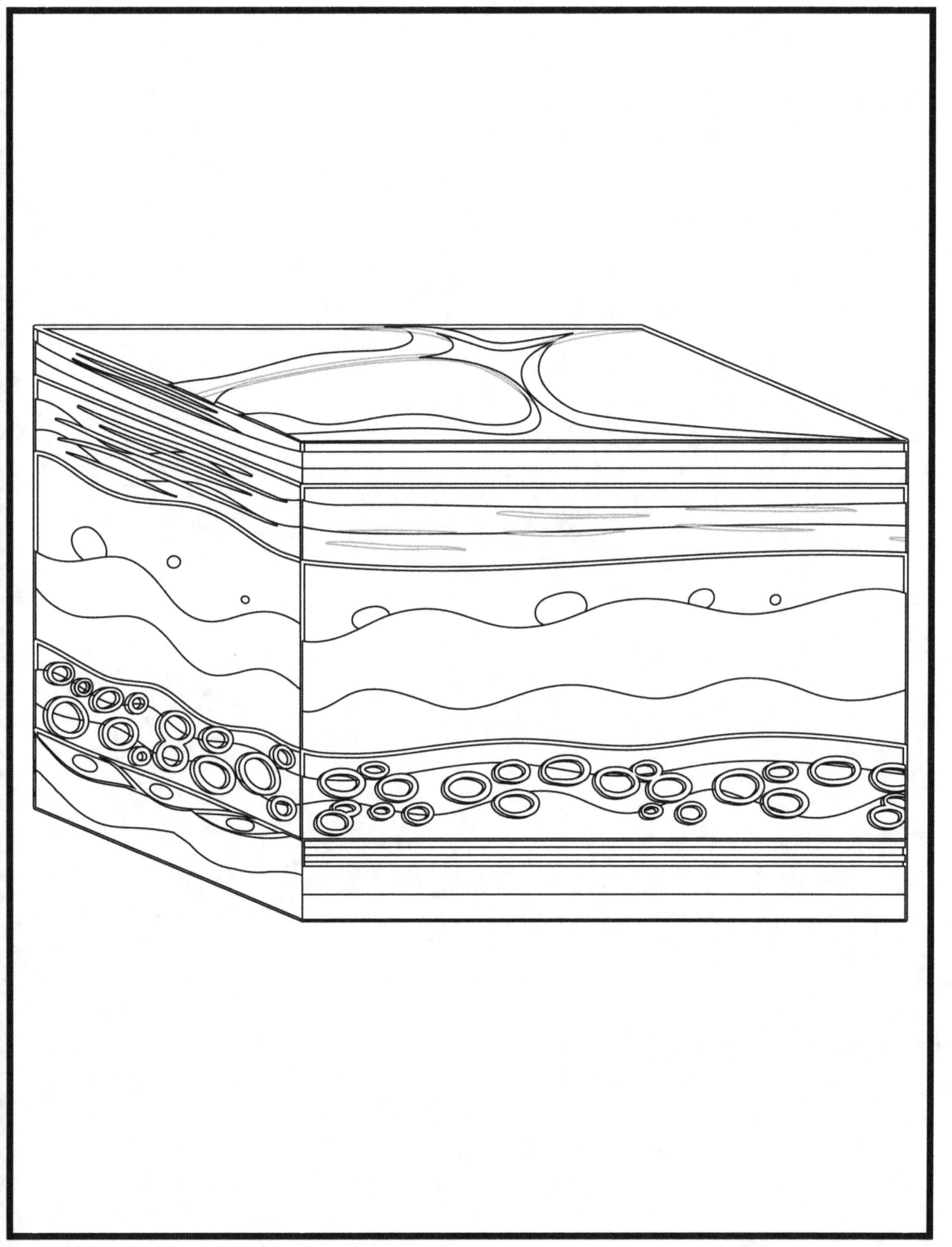

KNOWLEDGE MACHINE
OUR BRAIN
And Nervous System

The brain is where we do our thinking, all our senses are tied into our brain allowing ut to experience the outside world, we remember, have emotions , solve problems , worry about stuff, dream and we controle our bodies in our brain.

The nervous system is made up of the brain spinal cord and a large network of nerves that covers all parts of our body, together the nervous system helps deffernt parts of our body to communicate and allows our brain to controle what is going on.

Fun Facts

✦ Multitasking is impossible.

✦ An adult brain weighs about 3 pounds.

✦ about 75% of the brain is made up of water

✦ there is a nervous system for controlling the body at rest

✦ the human body has billions of nerve cells

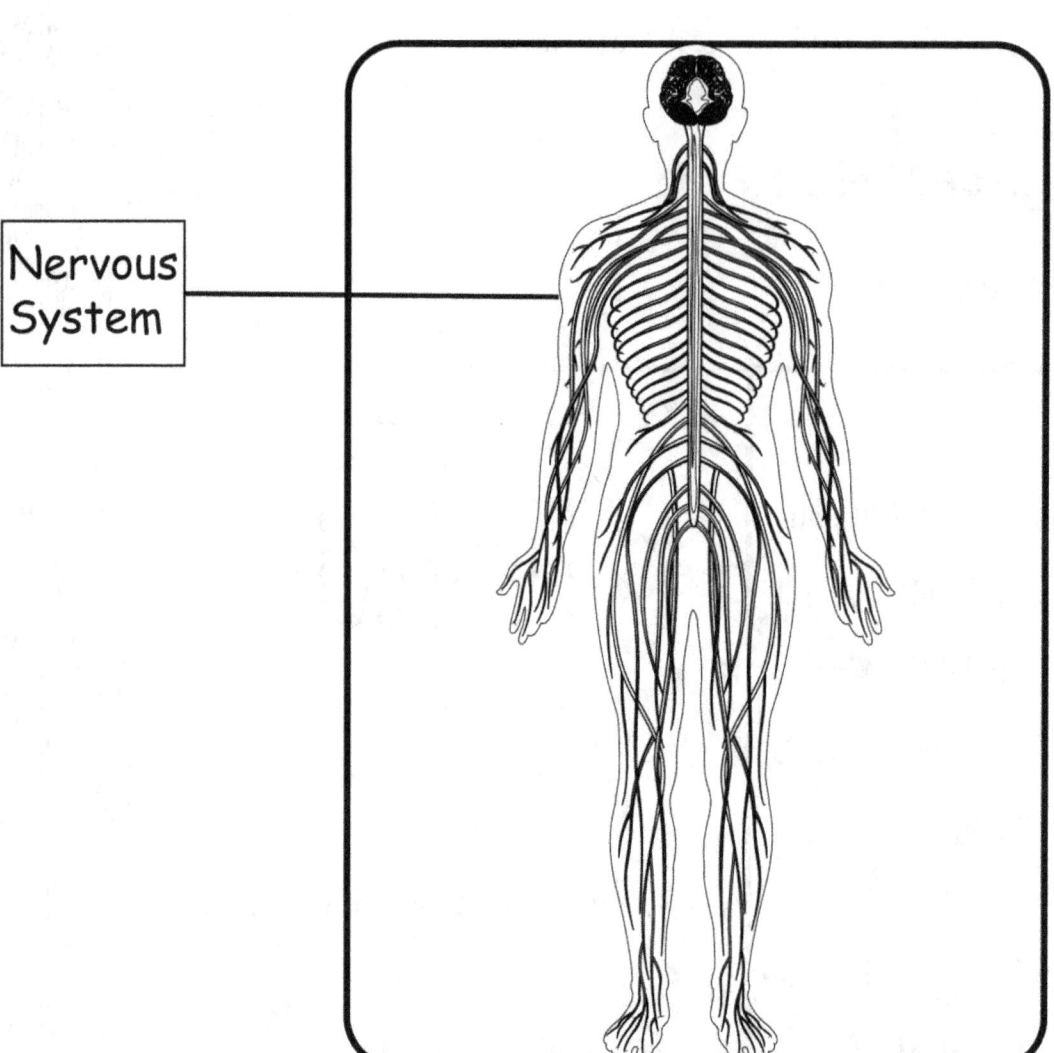

Nervous
System

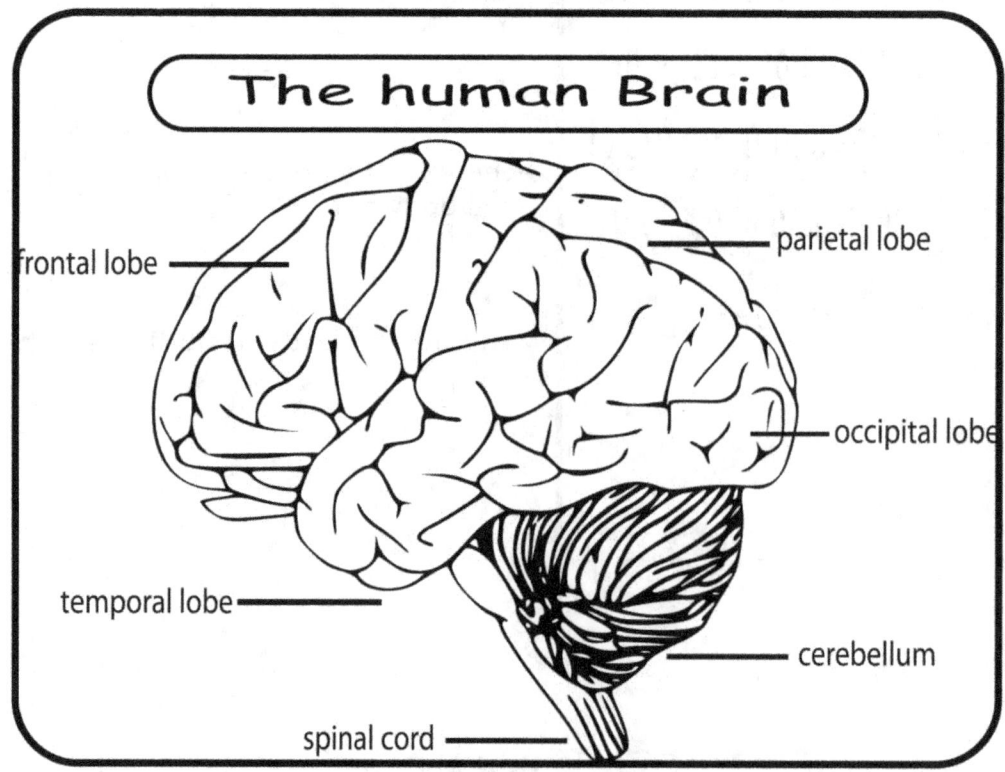

The human Brain

frontal lobe

parietal lobe

occipital lobe

temporal lobe

cerebellum

spinal cord

ACTIVITY

*Find these words and complete this word search puzzle

-Eye /-Disease /-Arms /-Organs /-Cells /-Blood /-Brain /-Ear
-Senses /-Nervous system /-Skin /-Taste /-Smell /-Spine
-Bones /-Digestion /-Muscles /-Heart /-Breathing /-Immunity

Q	X	S	E	E	S	A	E	S	I	D	R	I	W	X	N	A	B
Z	L	L	F	U	M	L	U	O	G	L	J	P	X	T	E	K	B
V	S	Z	Z	R	V	S	P	I	N	E	I	T	A	B	R	U	Y
R	Z	X	M	X	S	S	K	I	H	W	P	U	E	B	V	H	M
K	T	E	Y	E	E	W	Z	Q	Q	M	N	S	E	H	O	A	B
W	X	L	J	T	O	B	M	V	W	Q	W	M	O	C	U	N	R
R	T	E	S	Z	R	H	F	Y	Y	Z	W	R	G	Y	S	X	E
Y	E	A	L	A	S	E	N	S	E	S	G	A	S	M	S	H	A
P	T	O	I	Z	S	T	Q	Q	M	A	A	I	B	D	Y	E	T
E	X	N	N	M	D	G	J	U	N	X	B	A	D	O	S	Y	H
I	C	Q	E	O	L	P	S	S	B	X	V	H	J	O	T	P	I
M	C	L	A	O	I	C	O	S	L	W	I	O	A	L	E	A	N
M	L	C	P	A	L	T	S	T	L	L	W	R	A	B	M	G	G
U	P	X	V	E	B	H	S	S	C	L	E	V	L	Q	R	X	M
N	A	Q	S	N	K	L	E	E	M	D	Z	C	B	V	S	J	W
I	F	C	Z	E	J	I	Y	A	G	V	Z	O	N	I	K	S	E
T	B	O	N	E	S	X	Z	G	R	I	S	M	S	P	L	J	A
Y	R	I	V	G	M	G	D	B	T	T	D	H	Q	T	K	N	R

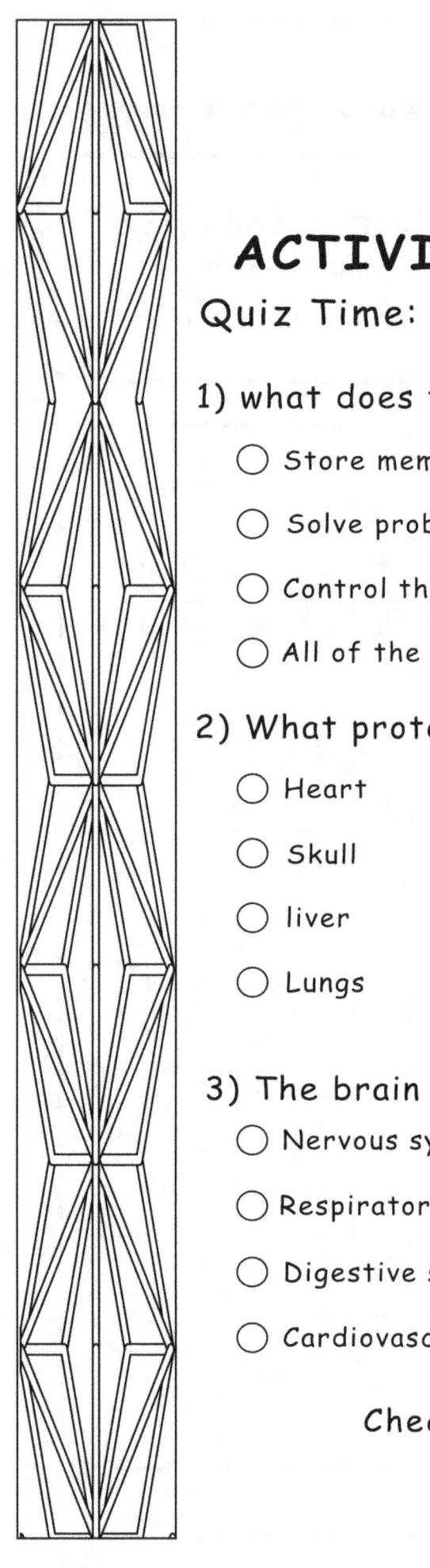

ACTIVITY

Quiz Time:

1) what does the brain do?

- ◯ Store memories
- ◯ Solve problems
- ◯ Control the body
- ◯ All of the above

2) What protects the brain?

- ◯ Heart
- ◯ Skull
- ◯ liver
- ◯ Lungs

3) The brain is part of which system?

- ◯ Nervous system
- ◯ Respiratory system
- ◯ Digestive system
- ◯ Cardiovascular system

Check the right answer with (x)

Coloring and Activity

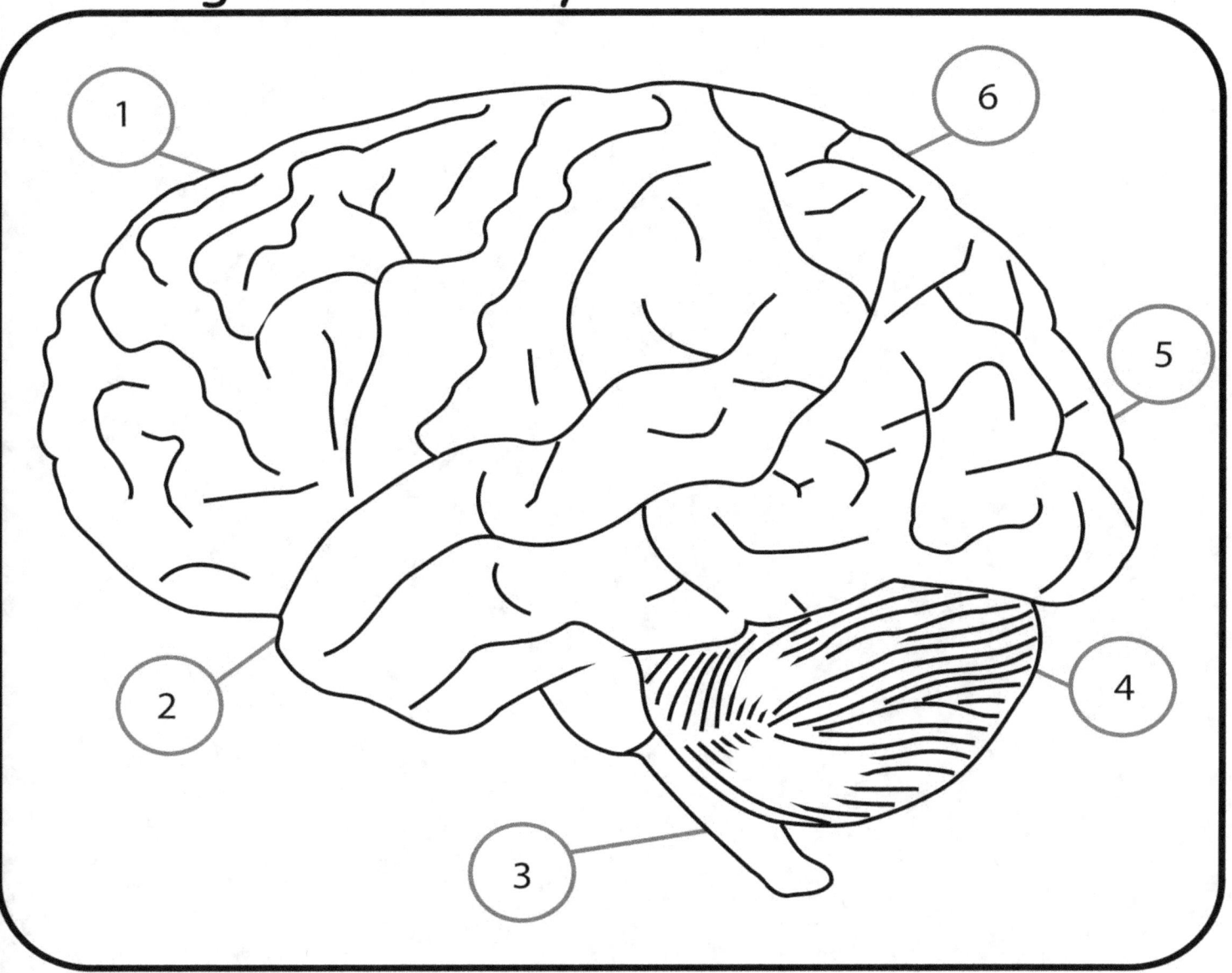

*connect each number with the right answer

①   temporal lobe

②   parietal lobe

③   frontal lobe

④   cerebellum

⑤   spinal cord

⑥   occipital lobe

SMELLS LIKE OUR NOSE

Smelling and tasting are two of the five senses. They often work together.

We use our nose to smell things. At the top of the inside of your nose are millions of tiny little hairs called cilia. These hairs are conncted to smell sensors which send signals to our brain about smell via the olfactory nerve. We smell things when they emit small molecules that float in the air and end up in our nose. We can't see these tiny molecules, but they are there. The reason we sniff is to get more of those molecules up into the top of our nose to where they can attach to the special sensors and determine the smell.
smelling helps us in many ways. It first makes our food taste better. We can't really taste that many flavors, but with the help of smell we can taste thousands of diffrent things. Also, smell helps to warn us from bad things like rotten food or smoke from fire.

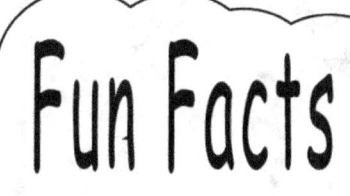

Fun Facts

✦ your nose contains your breath

✦ A sneeze can travel up to 99 miles per hour

✦ your nose can remember 50,000 diffrent scents

✦ it's impossibale to sneeze and open your eyes

✦ your nose humidifies the air you breathe

Human nose strecture

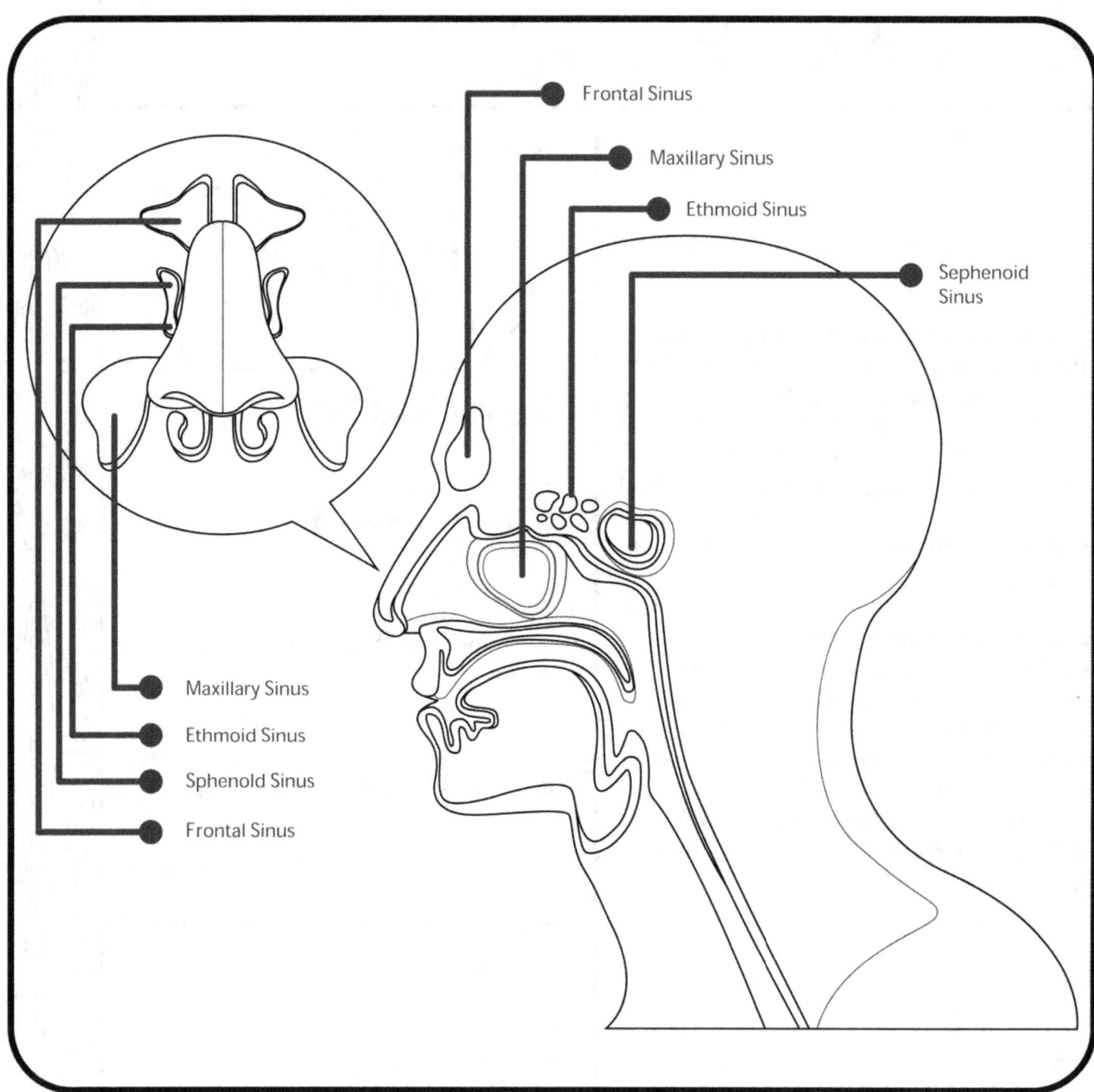

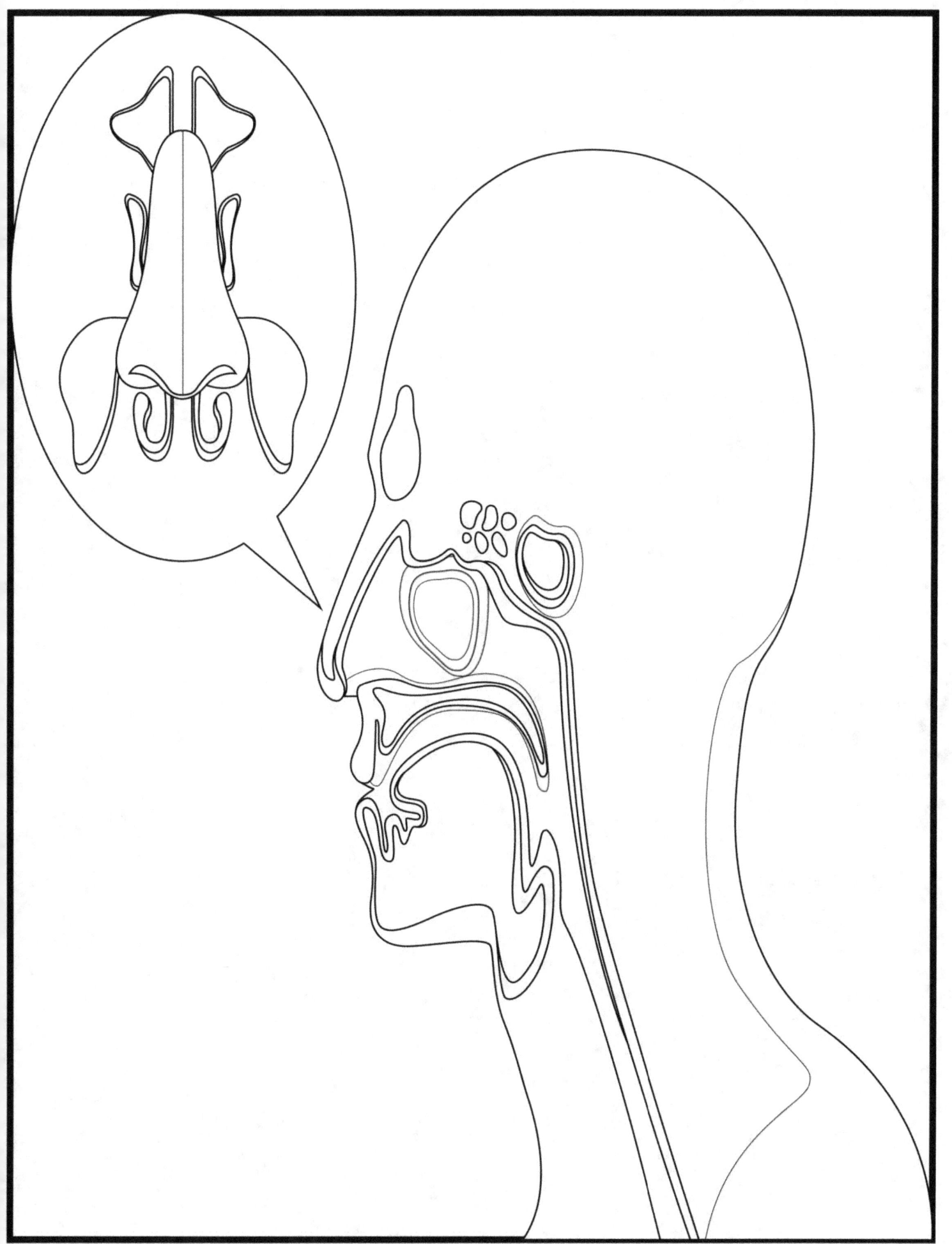

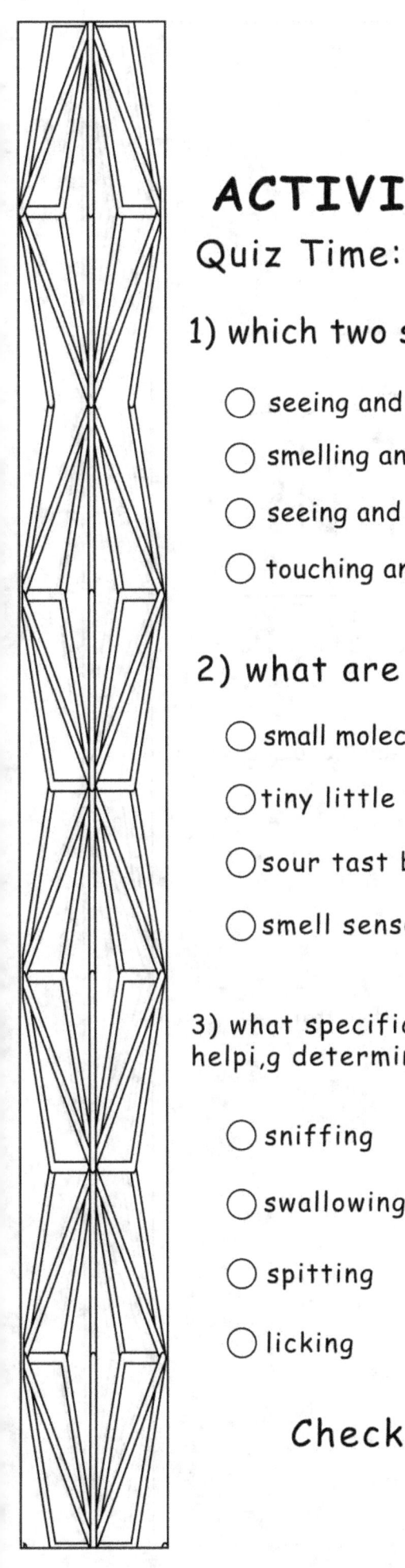

ACTIVITY
Quiz Time:

1) which two senses often works together?

- ◯ seeing and smelling
- ◯ smelling and tasting
- ◯ seeing and hearing
- ◯ touching and tasting

2) what are cillia?

- ◯ small molecules that float in the air into the nose
- ◯ tiny little hairs on the roof of the nose
- ◯ sour tast buds
- ◯ smell sensors in the nose which send signals to the brain

3) what specific action forces more molecules to travel up the nose, helpi,g determine the smell?

- ◯ sniffing
- ◯ swallowing
- ◯ spitting
- ◯ licking

Check the right answer with (x)

TASTY TONGUE

We use our tongue to taste things. The tongue uses taste buds or sensor cells to determine the type of food and send taste signals back to our brain. The tongue can taste four diffrent flavors, bitter, sour, salty and sweet. It was once thought that each of these tastes came from a diffrent spot on the tongue: sweet from the tip, salty from the sides, sour from the back sides, and bitter from the back. Now scientists say that flavors can be tasted from most any part of the tongue.

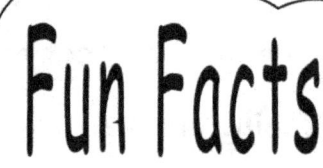

Fun Facts

◆ The tongue is about 3 inches long

◆ Tongue has between 2,000 and 4,000 taste buds

◆ you can't see your taste buds

◆ The tongue is not the strongest muscle in your body

Tongue Structure

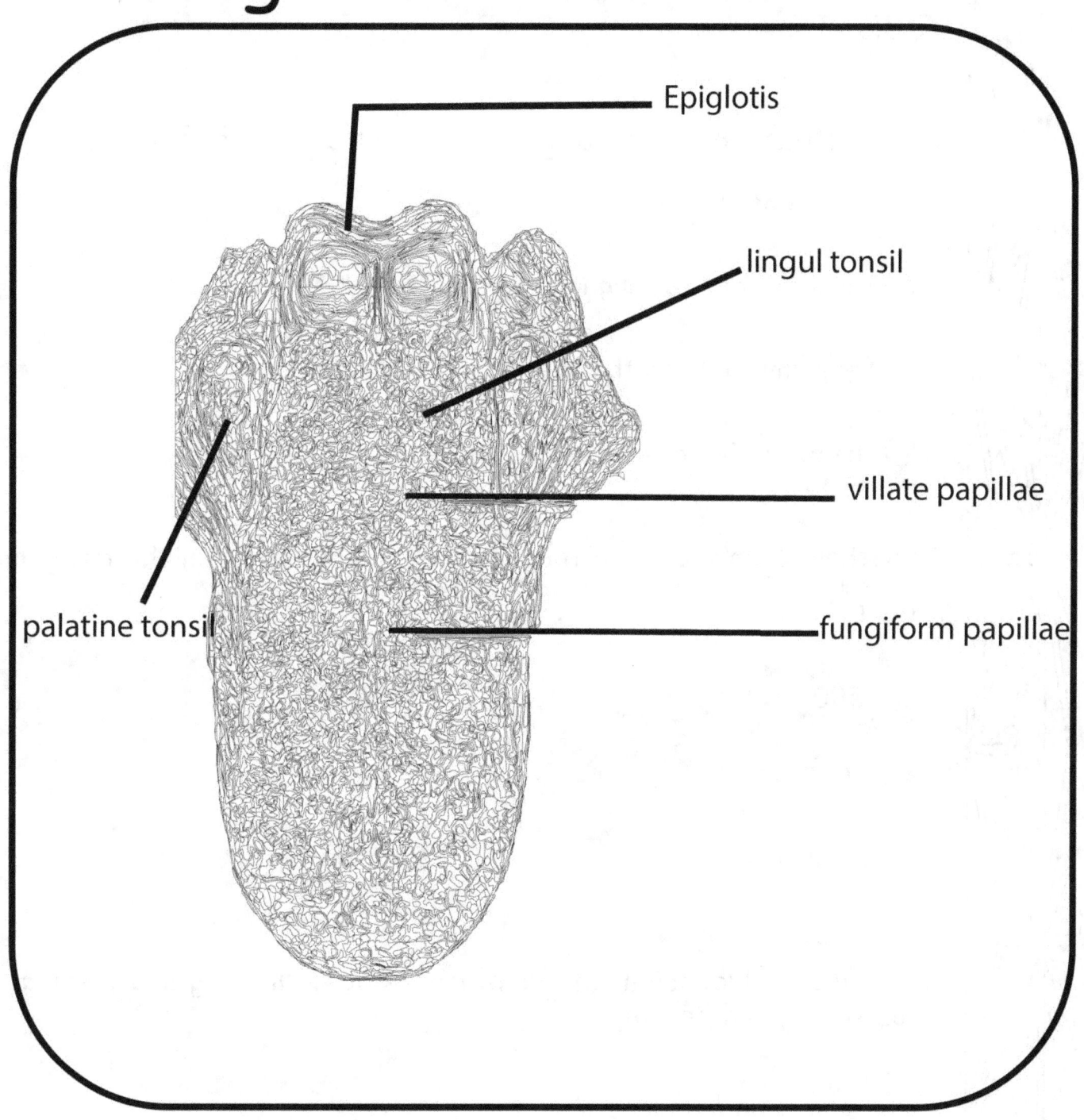

Epiglotis

lingul tonsil

villate papillae

palatine tonsil

fungiform papillae

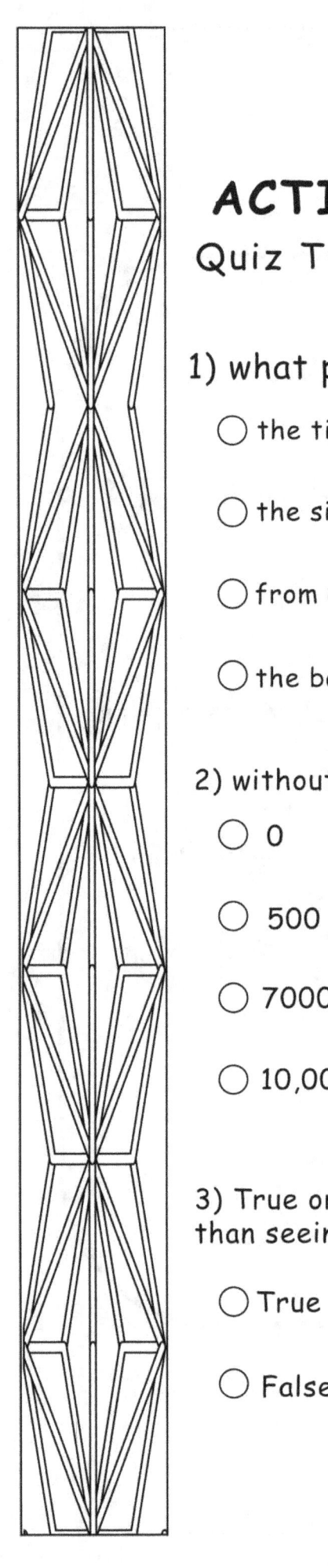

ACTIVITY

Quiz Time:

1) what part of the tongue can taste salty flavors?

○ the tip of the tongue

○ the sides of the tongue

○ from any parts of the tongue

○ the back of the tongue

2) without help from the tongue how many flavors can the nose smell?

○ 0

○ 500

○ 7000

○ 10,000

3) True or False: scientists konw more about smelling and tasting than seeing and hearing

○ True

○ False

Check the right answer with (x)

YOU SEE ME
OUR EYES

Sight is one of the five senses that help us to get information about what is going on into the world around us; We see through our eyes, which are organs that take in light and images and turn them electrical impulses that our brain can understand.

when we see something what we are seeing is actually reflected light, light rays bounce off of objects and into our eyes.

Fun Facts

- your eyes are about 1 inch across and weigh about 0.25 ounce

- the human eye can differentiate approximately 10 million different colors

- our eyes remain the same size throughout life

- the human eye blinks an average of 4.2 million times a year

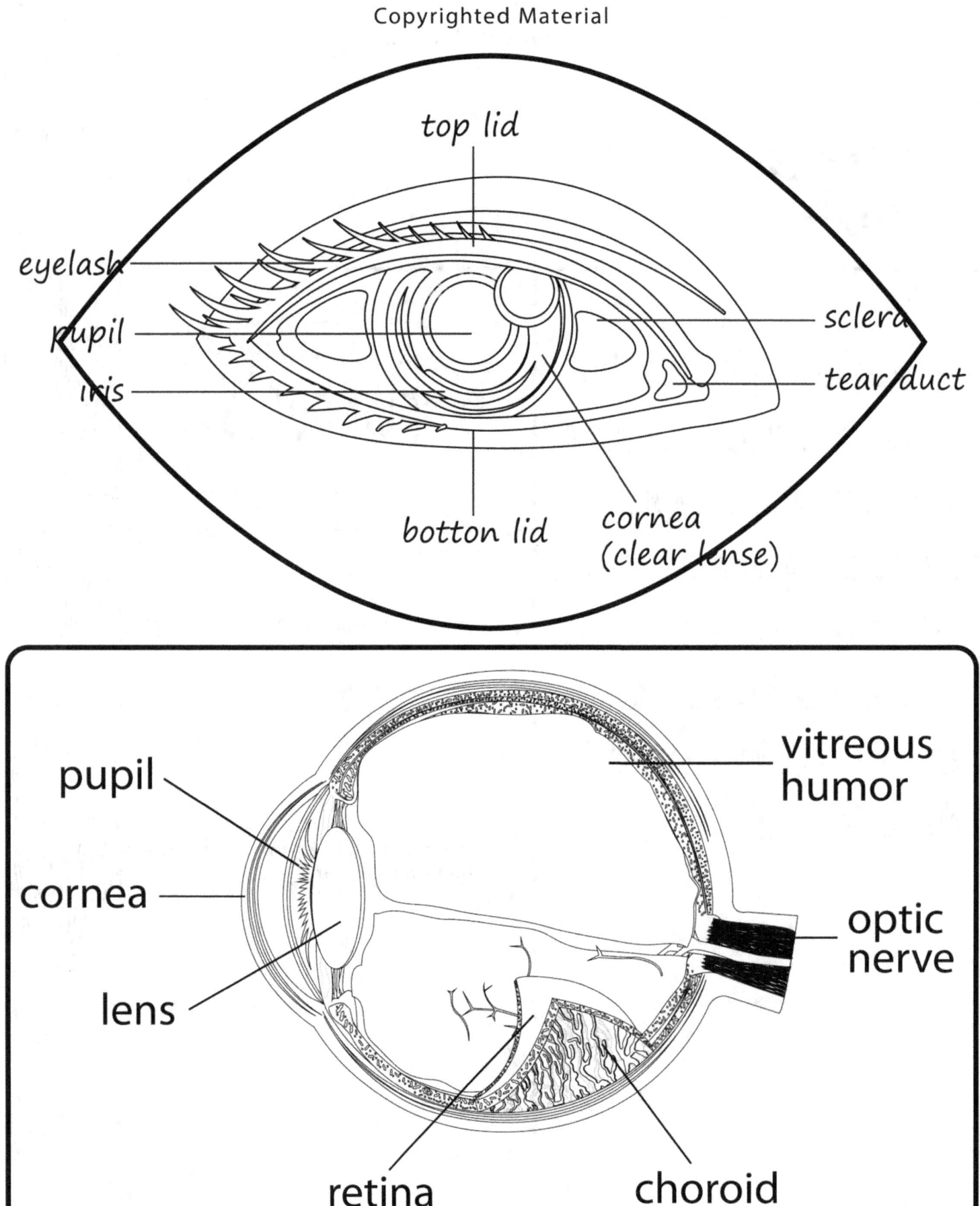

eyelash

pupil

iris

top lid

sclera

tear duct

botton lid

cornea
(clear lense)

pupil

cornea

lens

vitreous
humor

optic
nerve

retina

choroid

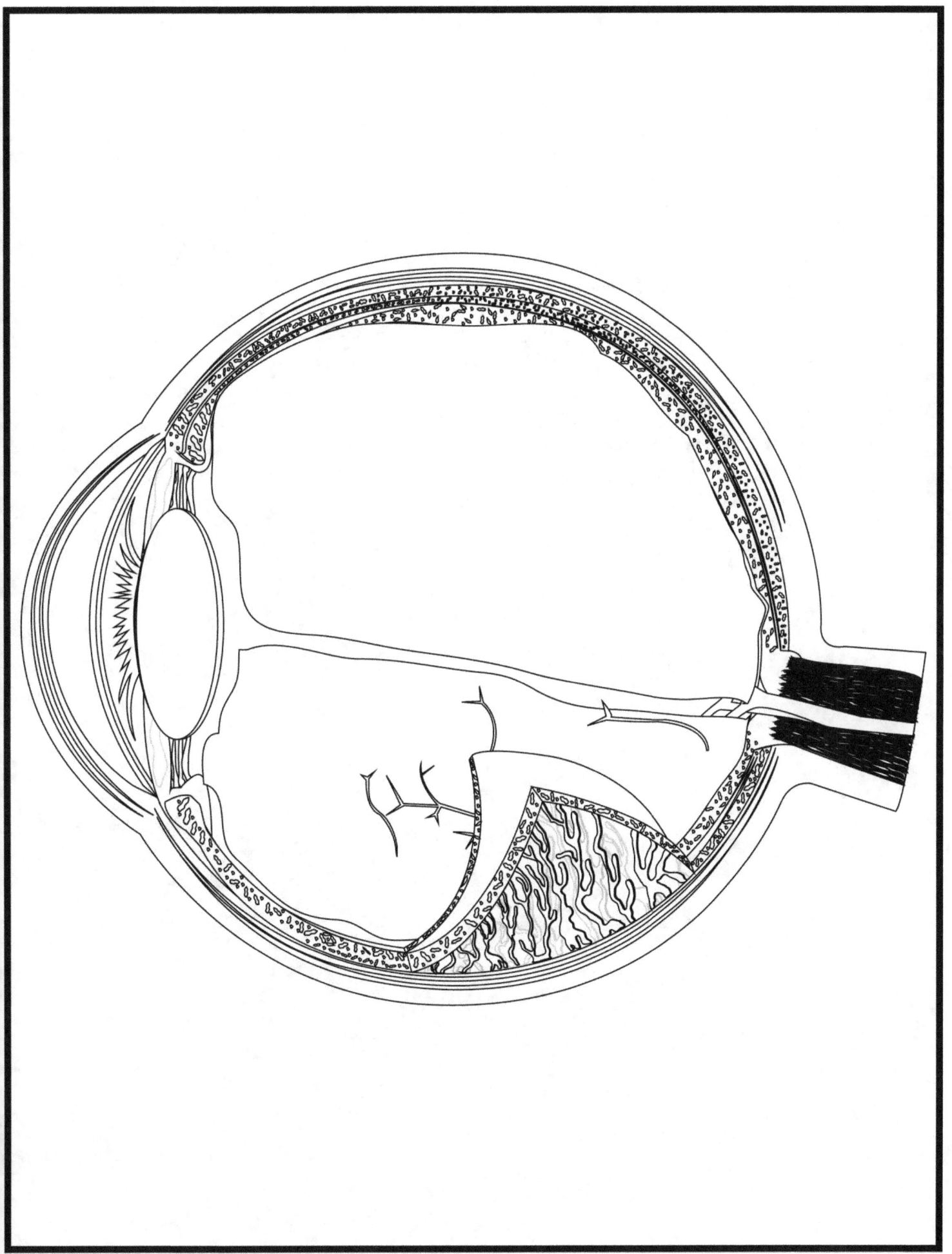

ACTIVITY

Quiz Time:

1) Our eyes are needed to perceive which of the five senses?

○ smell

○ taste

○ sight

○ touch

2) Wich of the following parts of the eye is the hole that lets in the light?

○ retina

○ lens

○ pupil

○ iris

3) the iris can change the _____ of the pupil.

○ color

○ shape

○ size

○ function

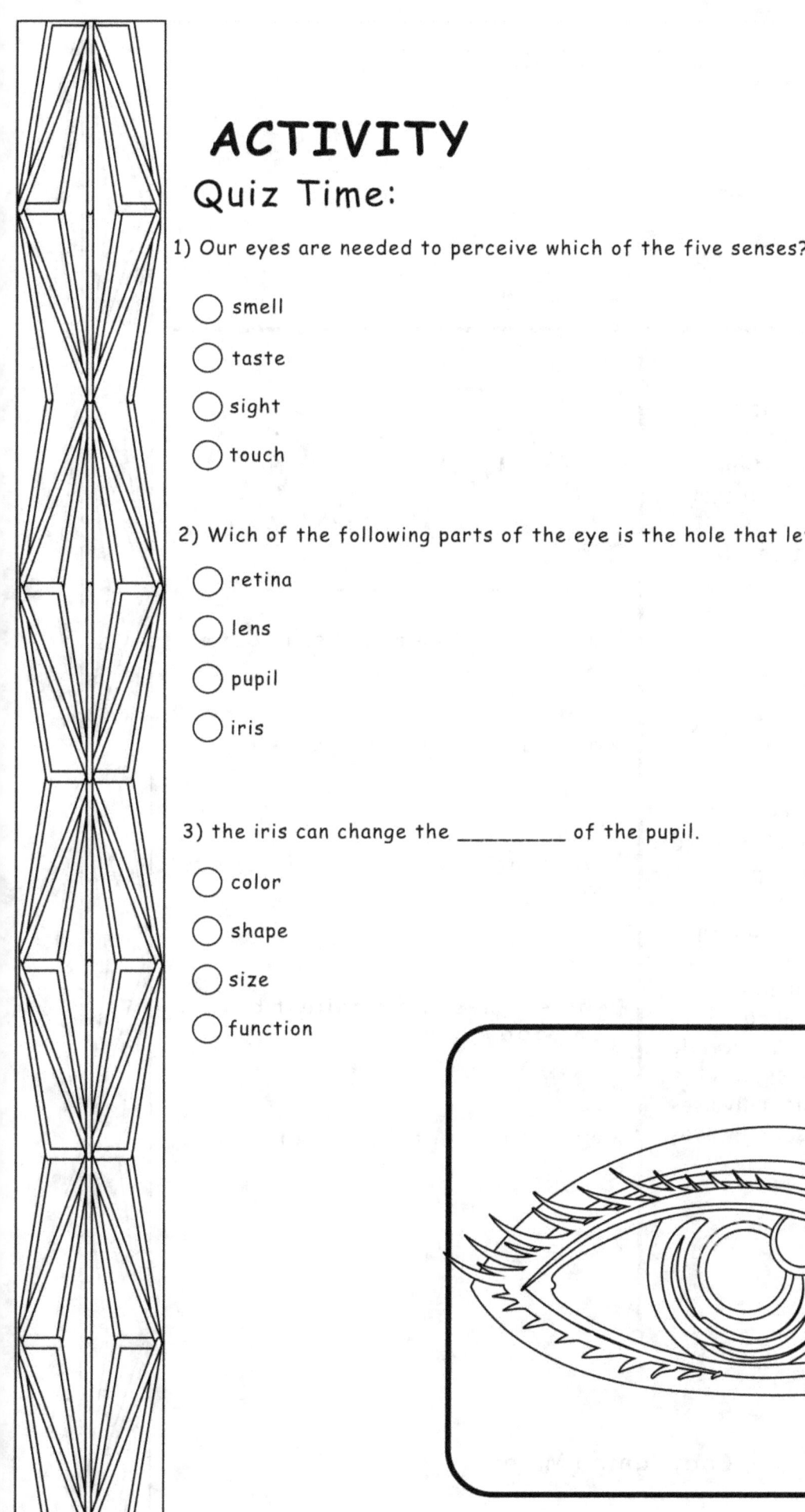

I HEAR YOU
OUR EARS

hearing is how we perceive sound. Its how our ear take sound waves and turn them into something our brain can understand
  there are three major parts of the ear that help us to gear
1/the outer ear and this one has three section:
-the pinna or auricle this is the part of the ear on the outside
-the ear canal this is a tube that helps sound to travel inside our ear
-the eardrum it is a thin sheet that vibrates when sound hits it
2/the middle ear: the middle ear is filled mostly with air and has three bones in it .
called ossicles they help you hear also called hammers,anvil, and stirrup. They amplify the or make it louder. The middle ear helps to transform sounds from the air to fluid inside the inner ear.
3/the inner ear: the inner ear is filled with fluid and has the hearing organ called the cochiea. This organ helps to take the vibrations and translate them into electrical signals for the nerve to sen to the brain. It actually uses little hairs that vibrate with the sound waves in the fluid. Then you hear it.

Fun Facts

◆ our sense of balance lies in our ears

◆ our ears are allways working

◆ we hear music better on our left side

◆ the ear has the smallest bone in our body

◆ wax is a natural protective agent

Ear strecture

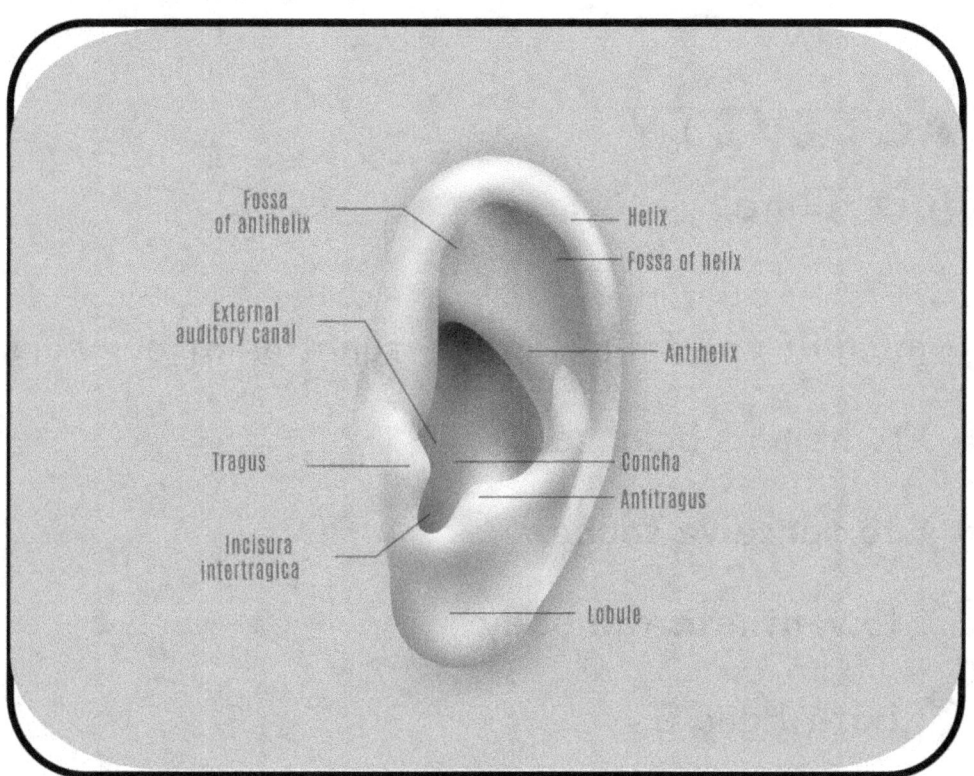

Fossa
of antihelix

Helix

Fossa of helix

External
auditory canal

Antihelix

Tragus

Concha

Antitragus

Incisura
intertragica

Lobule

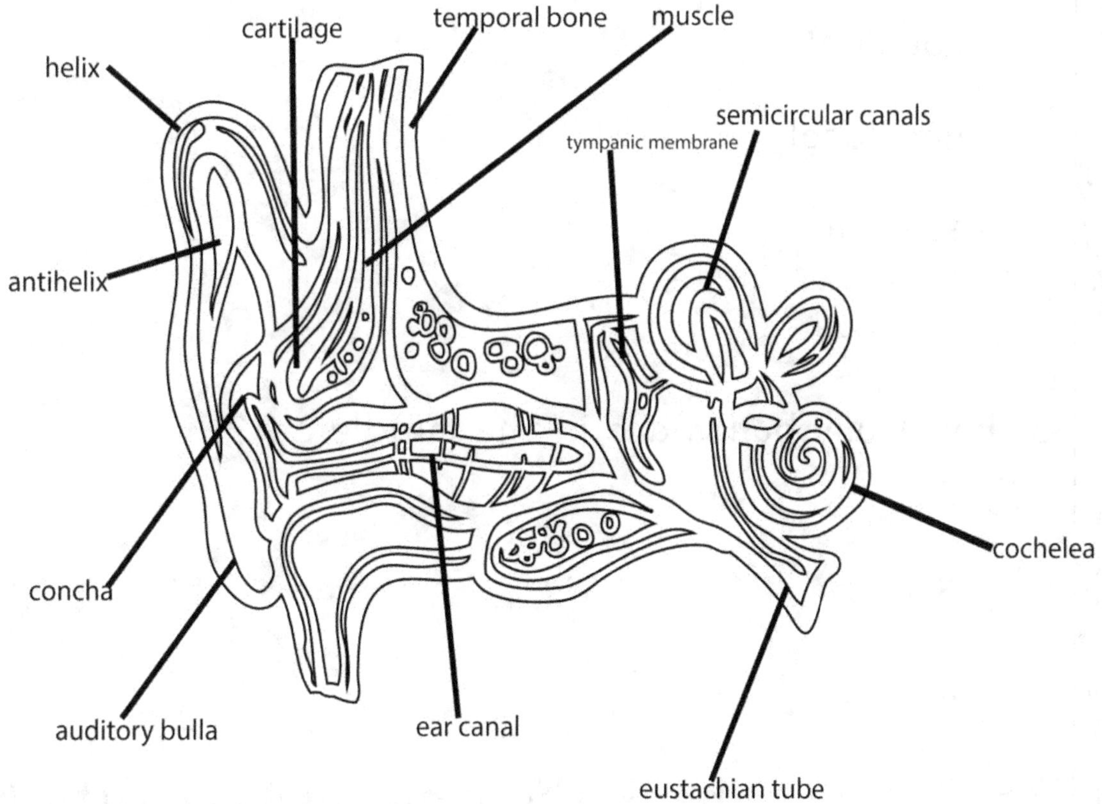

cartilage

temporal bone

muscle

helix

semicircular canals

tympanic membrane

antihelix

cochelea

concha

auditory bulla

ear canal

eustachian tube

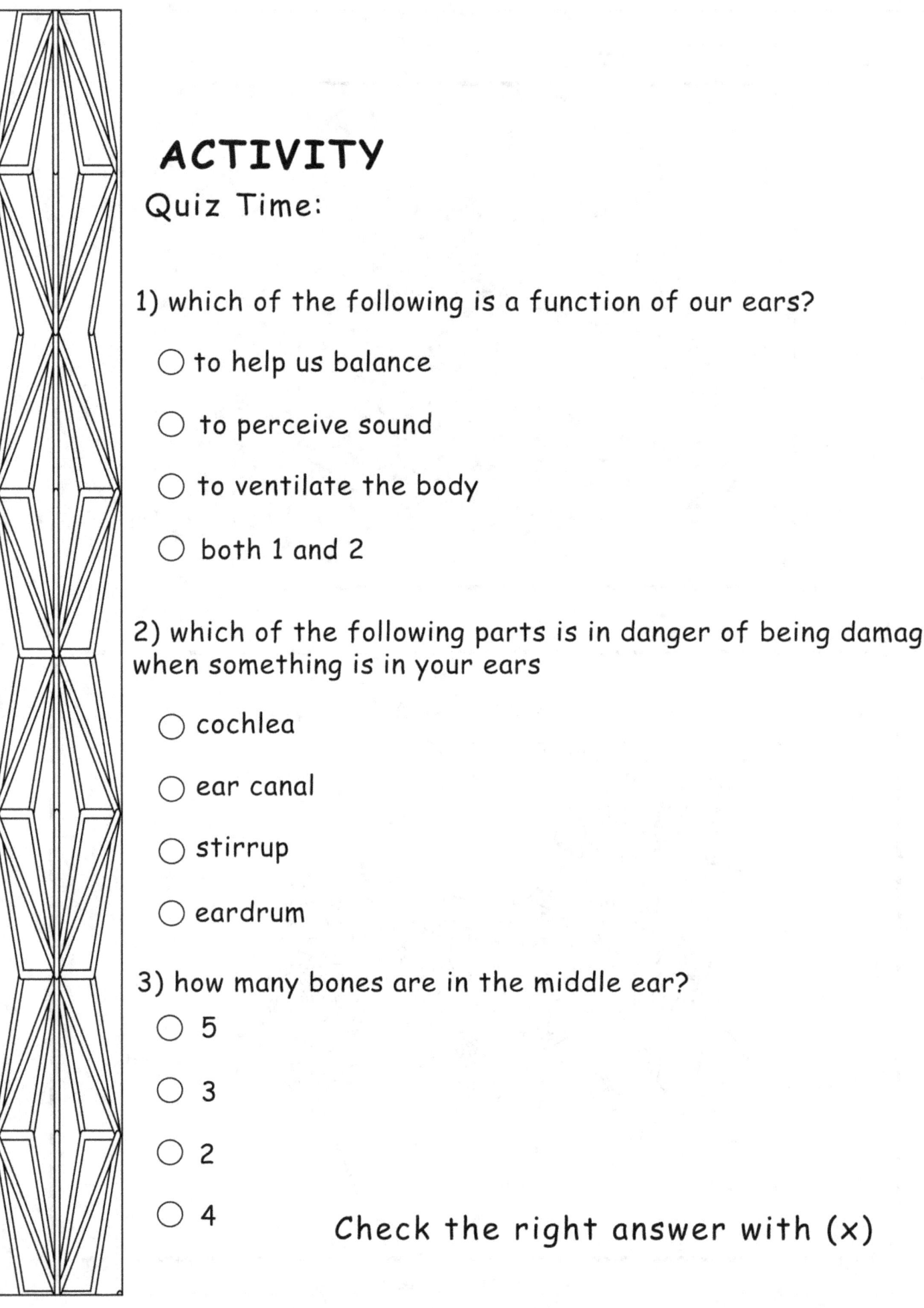

ACTIVITY

Quiz Time:

1) which of the following is a function of our ears?

○ to help us balance

○ to perceive sound

○ to ventilate the body

○ both 1 and 2

2) which of the following parts is in danger of being damaged when something is in your ears

○ cochlea

○ ear canal

○ stirrup

○ eardrum

3) how many bones are in the middle ear?

○ 5

○ 3

○ 2

○ 4

Check the right answer with (x)

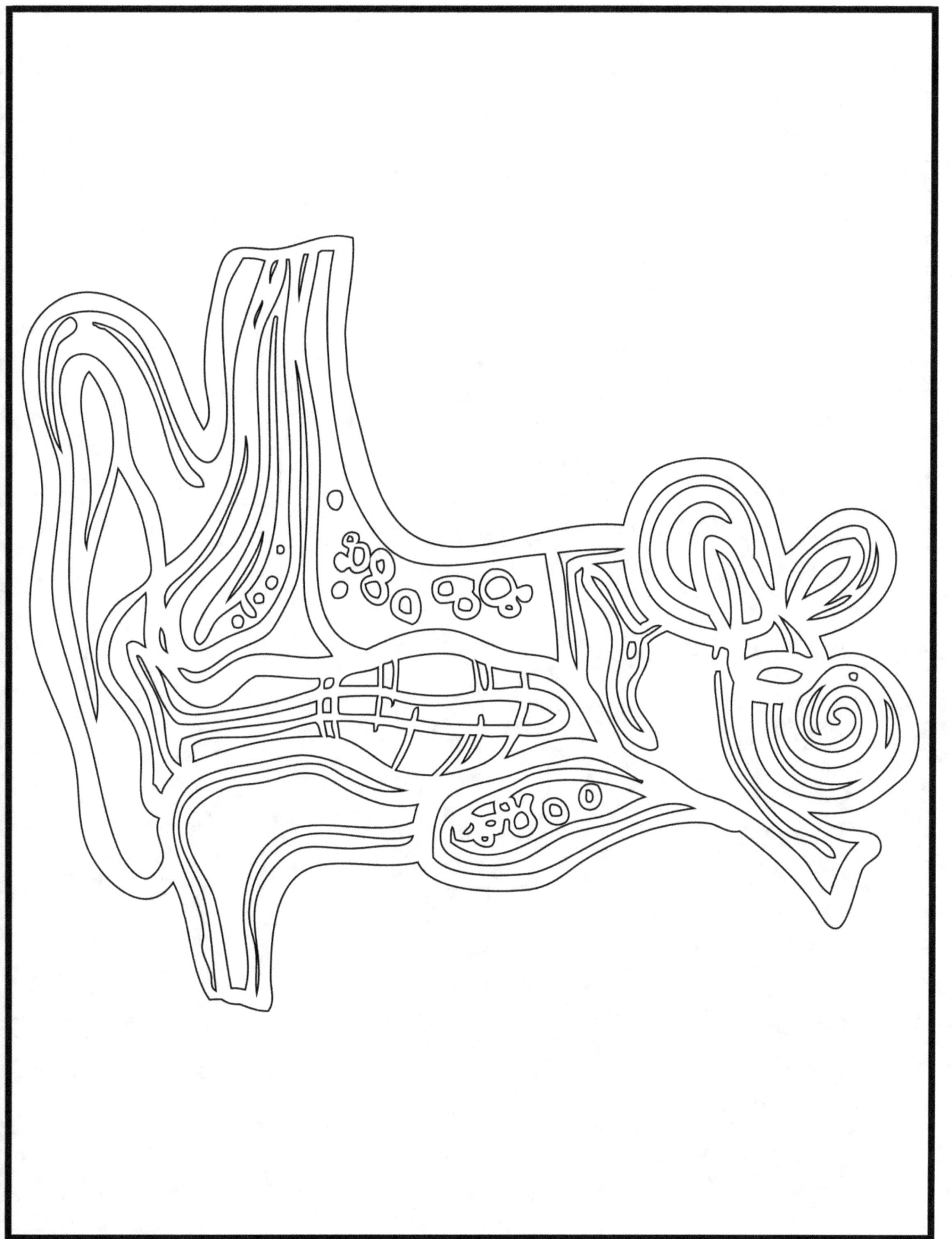

OUR DIEGESTIVE SYSTEM

Our body need food to provide it with energy, vitamins, and minerals. However in order use food, we must first break it down into substances that the various organs and cells in our body can use. This is the job of our digestive system.

The digestive system acts in stages to digest our food. Each stage is important and prepares the food for the next stage the entire length of our digestive system is around 20 to 30 feet.

the major steps of the digestive system:

1/chewing: chewing is the first stage of the digestive system. When you chew your food it breaks up bog pieces into little pieces that are easier to digest and swallow also, your saliva is more than just water. It has special enzymes in that start to break down starchy food while you chew.

2/ swallowing: it may seem like a simple process to us. It just sort of happens but food doesn't just fall down our throats into ourstomach. First, our tongue helps to push food into the back of the throat. Then there are special throat muscles that force the food down into a long tube that leads to our stomach, called the esphagus.

3/stomach: food hangs out in the stomach for around four hours. While the food sits there are more enzymes go to work on it breaking down things like proteins that our bodies can use.

4/small intestine: the first part of the small intestine works with juices from the liver and pancreas to continue to break down food.

5/large intestine: the last stage is the large intestine any food that the body doesn't need is sent to the large intestine and later leaves the body as waste.

Fun Facts

◆ the average person produces 2 pints of saliva every day.

◆ the muscles in your esophagus act like a giant wave.

◆ the second part of your small intestine is called the jejunum.

◆ enzymes in your digestive system are what separate food into the different nutrients that your body needs

Digestive System

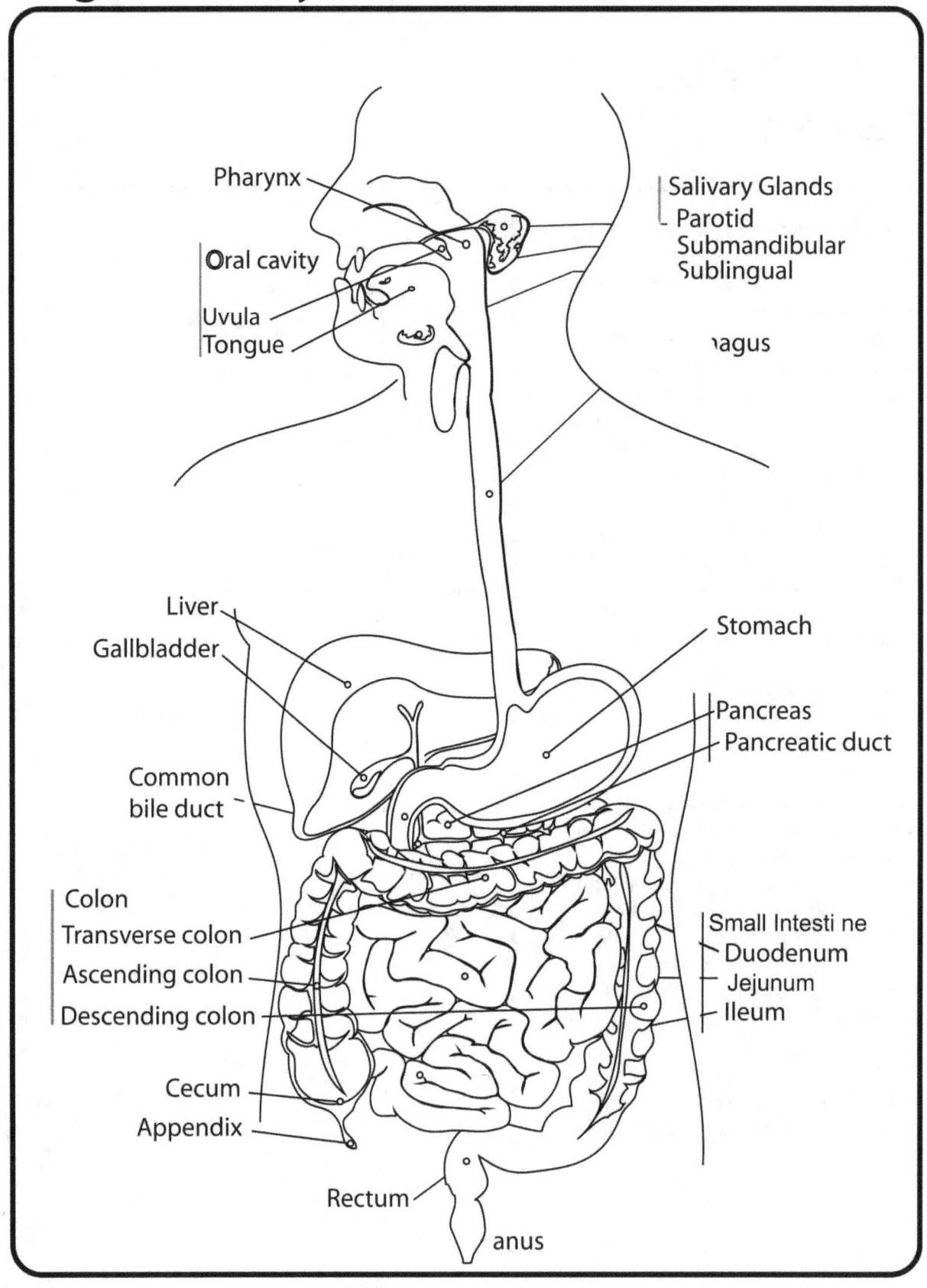

Pharynx

Oral cavity

Uvula
Tongue

Salivary Glands
Parotid
Submandibular
Sublingual

ıagus

Liver
Gallbladder

Stomach

Common
bile duct

Pancreas
Pancreatic duct

Colon
Transverse colon
Ascending colon
Descending colon

Small Intesti ne
Duodenum
Jejunum
Ileum

Cecum
Appendix

Rectum

anus

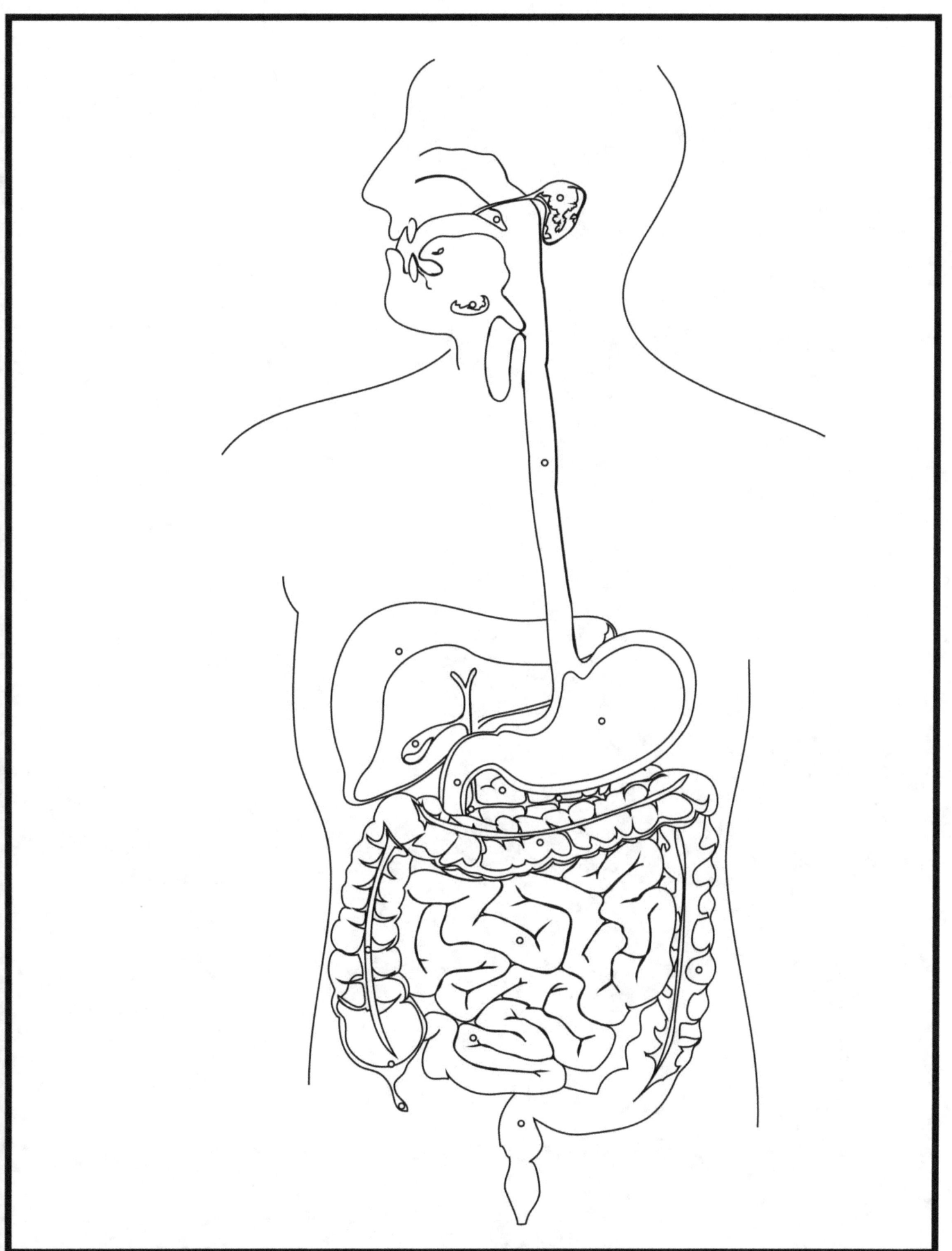

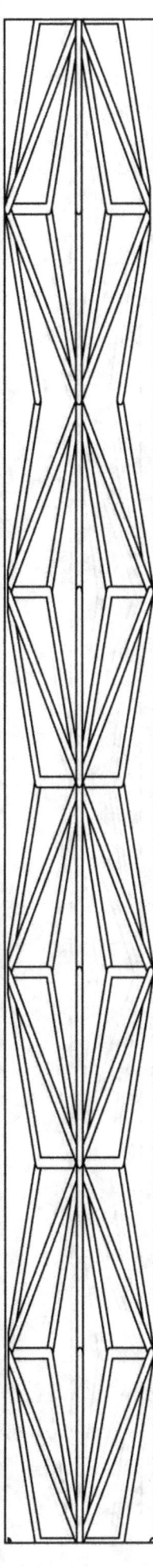

ACTIVITY
Quiz Time:

1) what's the main purpose of the digestive system?

⭕ to fight off diseases

⭕ to distribute enrgy throughout the body

⭕ to break down food

⭕ to regenerate cells

2) True or Flase: the digestive system is about 20 to 30 feet long?

⭕ True

⭕ False

3) what type of protein does saliva have to help break down food?

⭕ collagen

⭕ oxytocin

⭕ enzymes

⭕ insulin

Check the right answer with (x)

OUR HEART AND CIRCULATION

The heart is a large organ about the size of your fist. It sits in your rib cage just to the left of the center of your chest. The heart is made of a lot of muscles that pumps blood through our bodies. Veins blood to the the heart pumps back out again on arteries. The main artery leaving the heart is called aorta. In order for blodd not to go backwards, there are valves to make sure the blood only gets pumped in the correct direction There are four sets of valves in the heart.

The heart has two main pumps. One sends the blood throughout the body, while the other sends blood from veins up to the lungs to drop off carbon dioxide and pick up more oxygen. The heart beats at differnt rates depending on what the body is doing. If you are just sitting around, it will beat slowly. If you are runnig fast, the heart will beat faster to get oxygen to your muscles.

Blood circulates, constantly through our entire body, as it passes through our body it picks up nutrients from our food and drops them off the cells that need them. It alsi picks up oxygen drom our lungs and drops it off at cells to be used for energy. The blood then picks up waste carbon dioxide from the cells and drops it off the lungs for us to breathe back out.

Fun Facts

◆ there are four main blood types: A, B, O and AB

◆ Your heart will beat about 115,000 times each day

◆ your heart pumps about 2,000 gallons of blood every day

◆ an electrical system controls the rhythm of your heart

◆ if the red blood cells fromone person were to be stacked in the sky they would reach 31,000 miles

Heart strecture

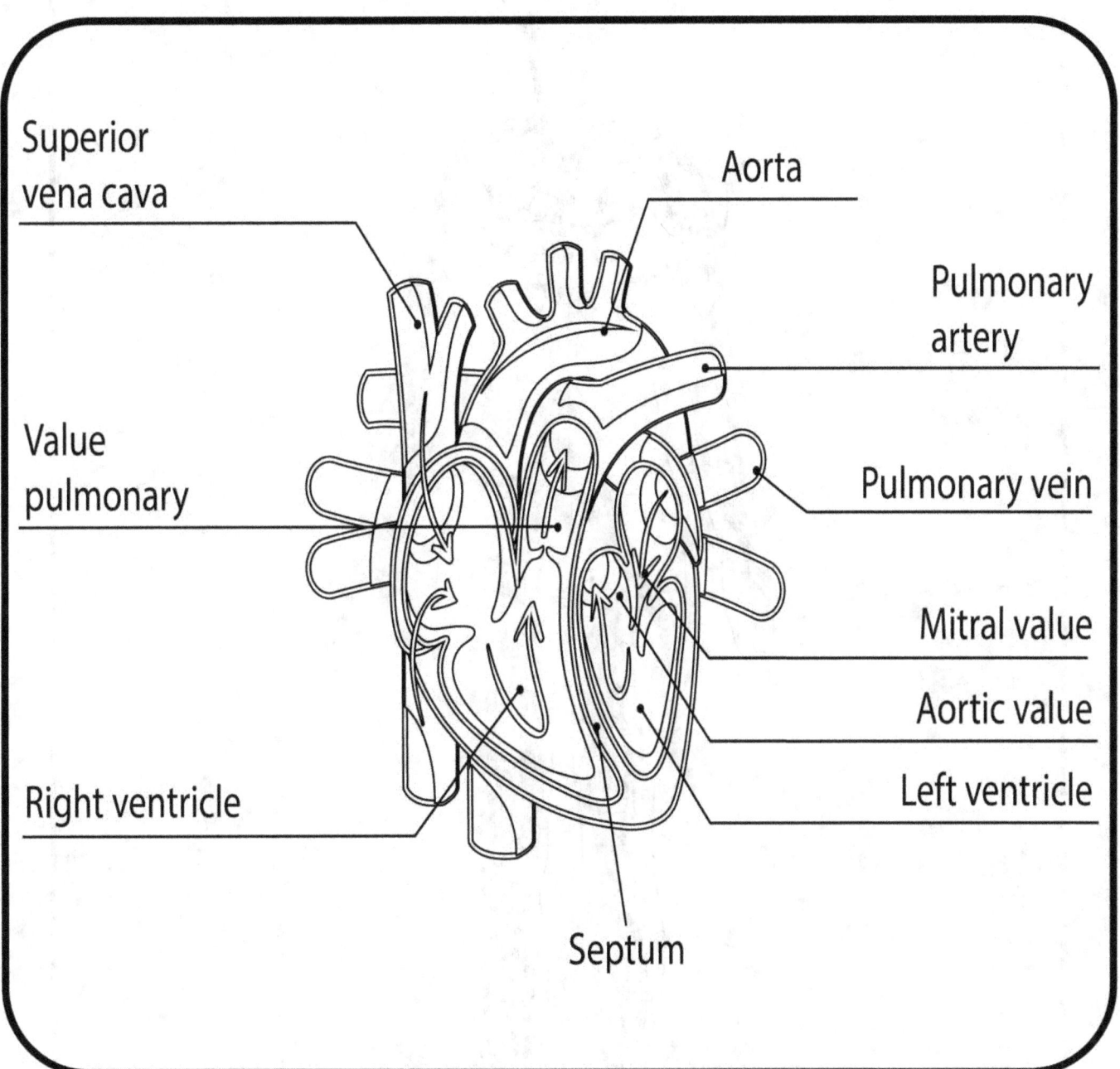

Superior
vena cava

Aorta

Pulmonary
artery

Value
pulmonary

Pulmonary vein

Mitral value

Aortic value

Right ventricle

Left ventricle

Septum

Circulatory system

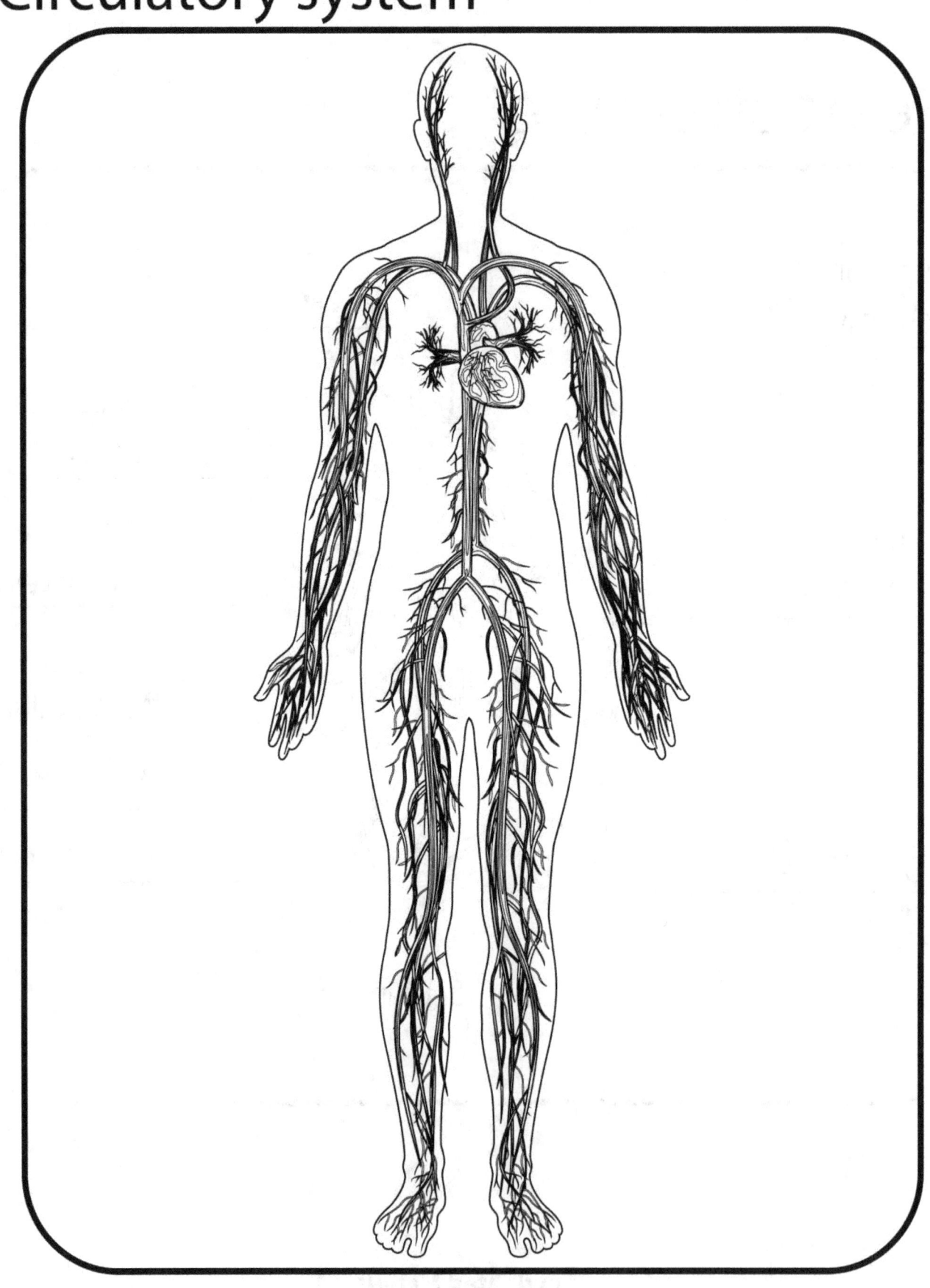

Heart Blood Flow

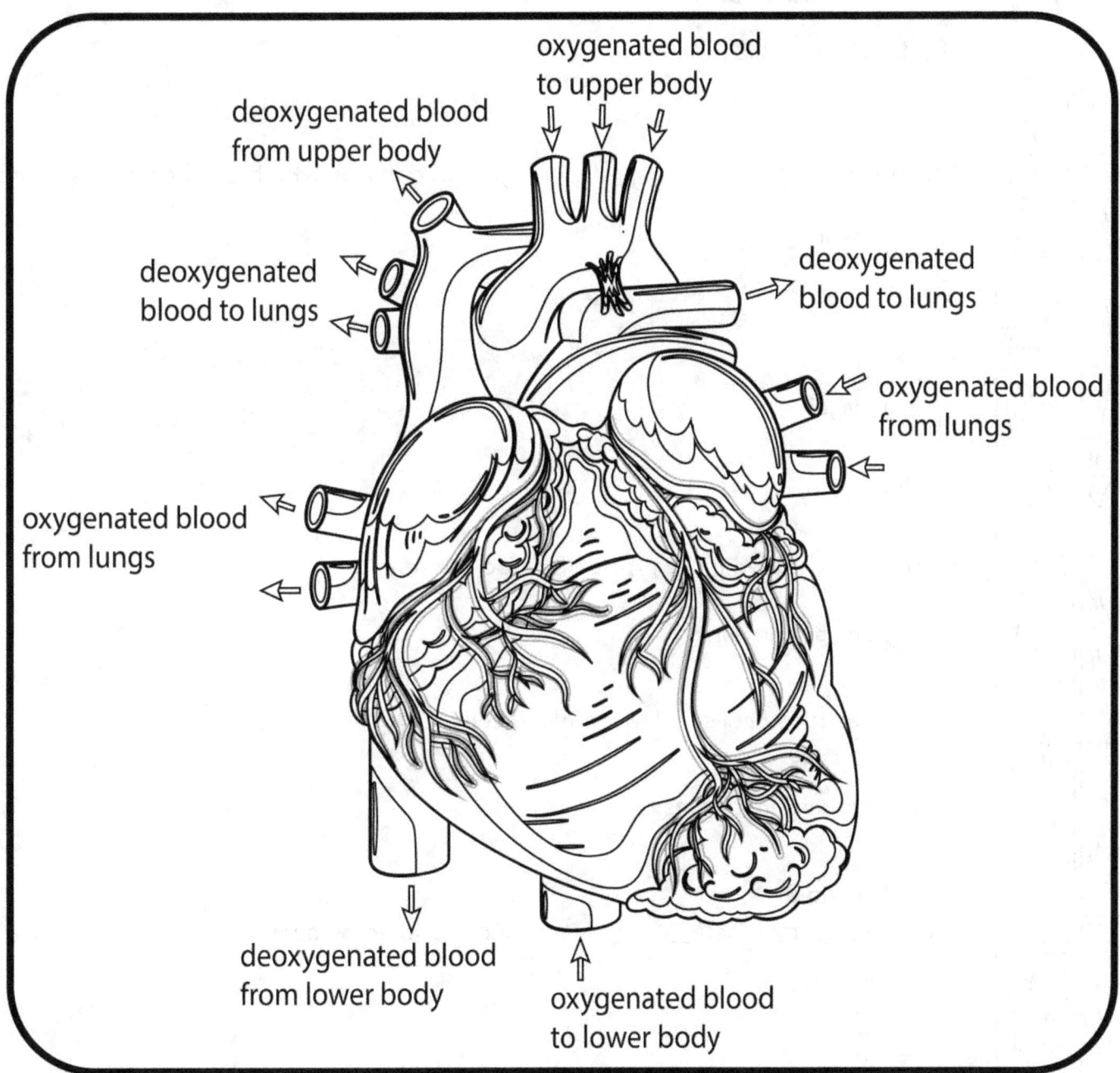

oxygenated blood
to upper body

deoxygenated blood
from upper body

deoxygenated
blood to lungs

deoxygenated
blood to lungs

oxygenated blood
from lungs

oxygenated blood
from lungs

deoxygenated blood
from lower body

oxygenated blood
to lower body

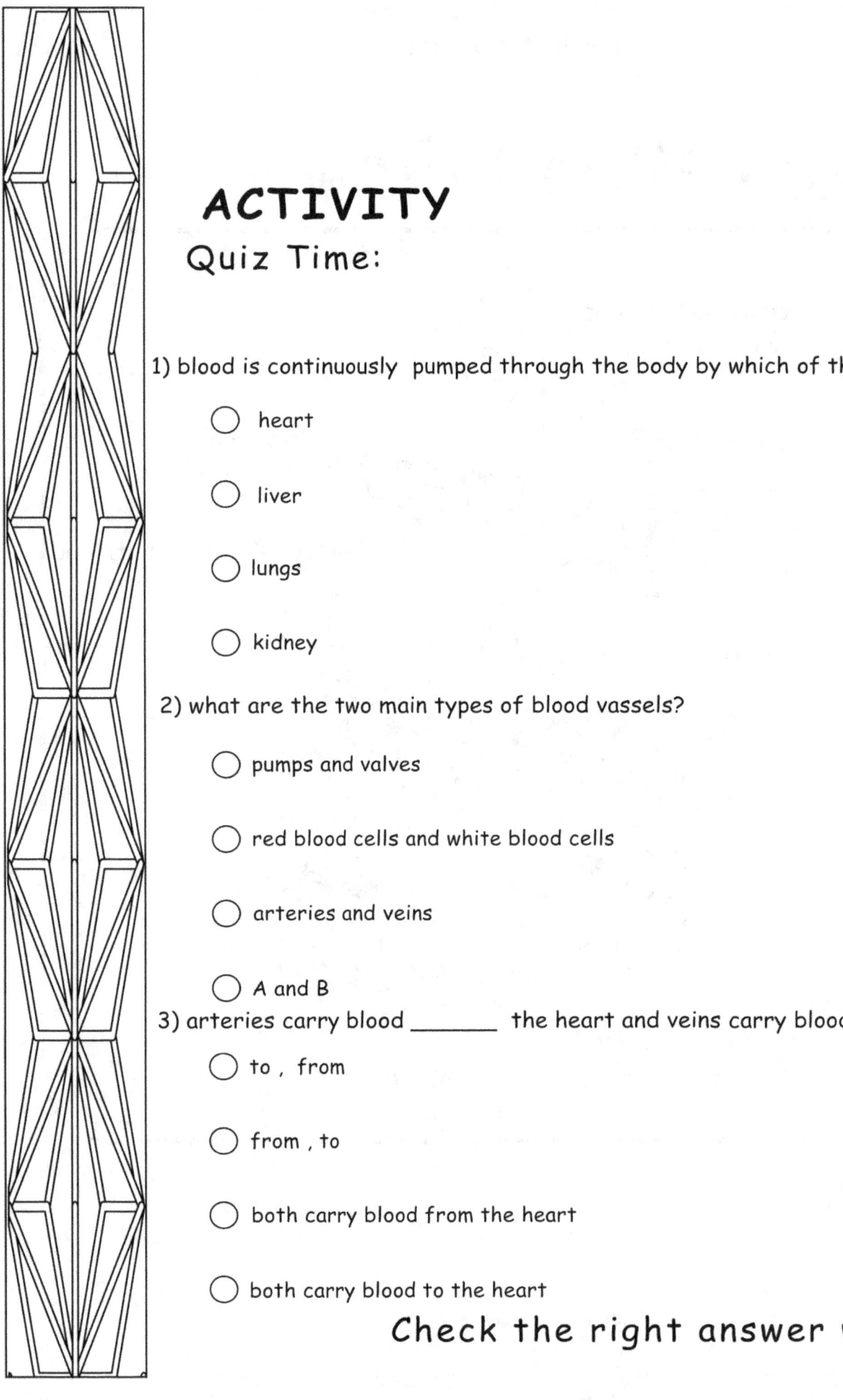

ACTIVITY
Quiz Time:

1) blood is continuously pumped through the body by which of the following organs

○ heart

○ liver

○ lungs

○ kidney

2) what are the two main types of blood vassels?

○ pumps and valves

○ red blood cells and white blood cells

○ arteries and veins

○ A and B

3) arteries carry blood _____ the heart and veins carry blood _____ the hea

○ to , from

○ from , to

○ both carry blood from the heart

○ both carry blood to the heart

Check the right answer with (x)

Color the heart and name the areas selected

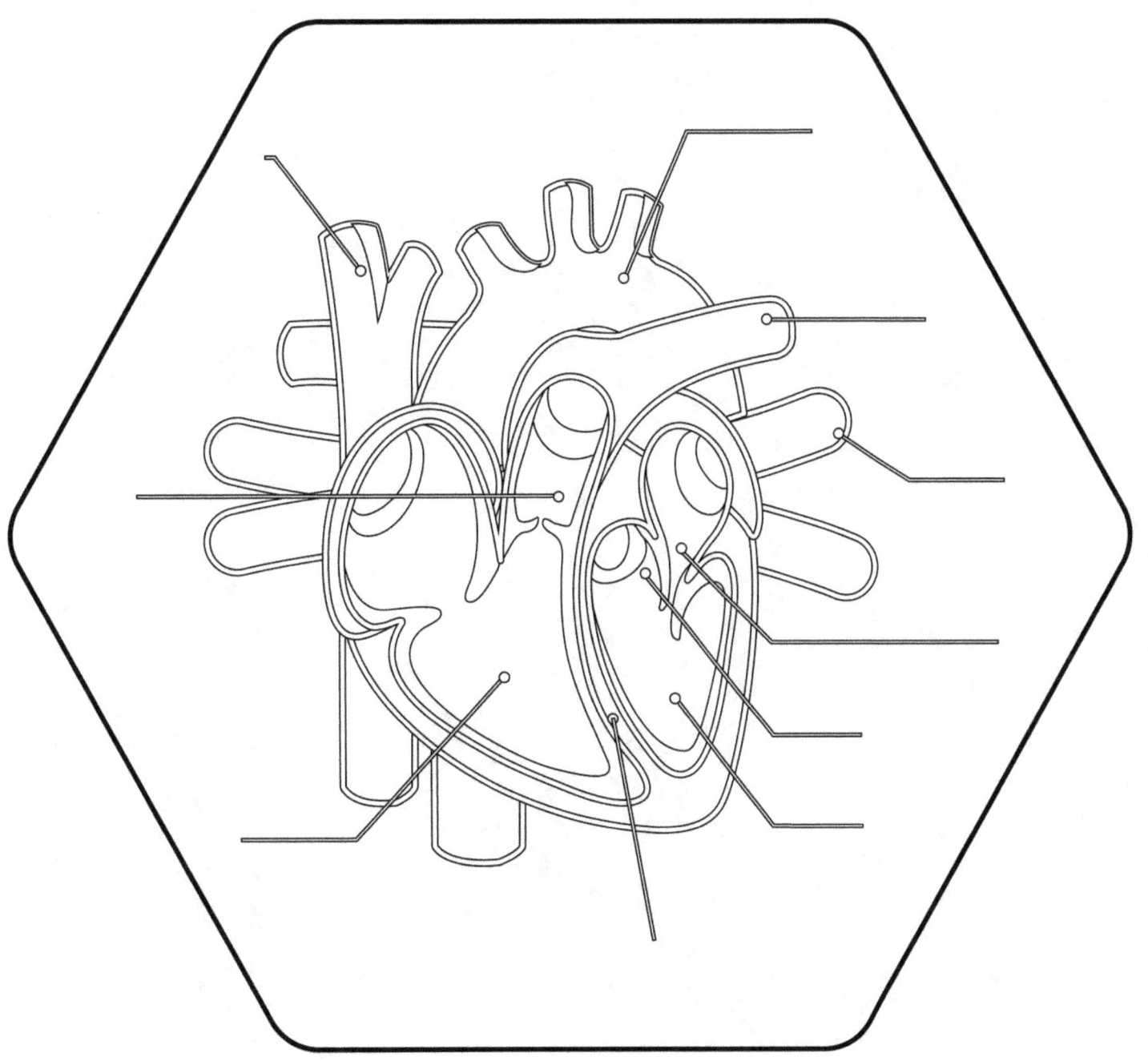

BREATHING OUR LUNGS AND RESPIRATORY SYSTEM

The lungs are the primary organs of the respiratory system in humans and many other animals including a few fish and some snails. In mammals and most other vertebrates, two lungs are located near the backbone on either side of the heart. Their function in the repiratory system is to extract oxygen from the atmosphere and transfer it into the bloodstream, and to release carbon dioxide from the bloodstream into the atmosphere, in a process of gas exchange. Respiration is driven by different muscular systems in different species.

Humans breathe through something the respiratory system. This system is made up primarily of our lungs and windpipe.

Our body is a very complex system. One of the main things it needs is energy. When we eat our body digests the food to get complex molecules like glucose, which it can use for energy. However, food alone isn't enaugh. The cells also need oxygen to react with the glucose to creat the energy. We get the oxygen to our cells with the respiratory system and by breathing.

Fun Facts

◆ A person usually breaths an average of 13 pints of air every minute.

◆ Lungs aren't the same size to accommodate the heart, the right lung is larger than the left lung

◆ Lungs float on water

◆ Lungs and tennis courts can be the same size

◆ Oxygen anly plays a small part in breathing

Humans
Respiratory System

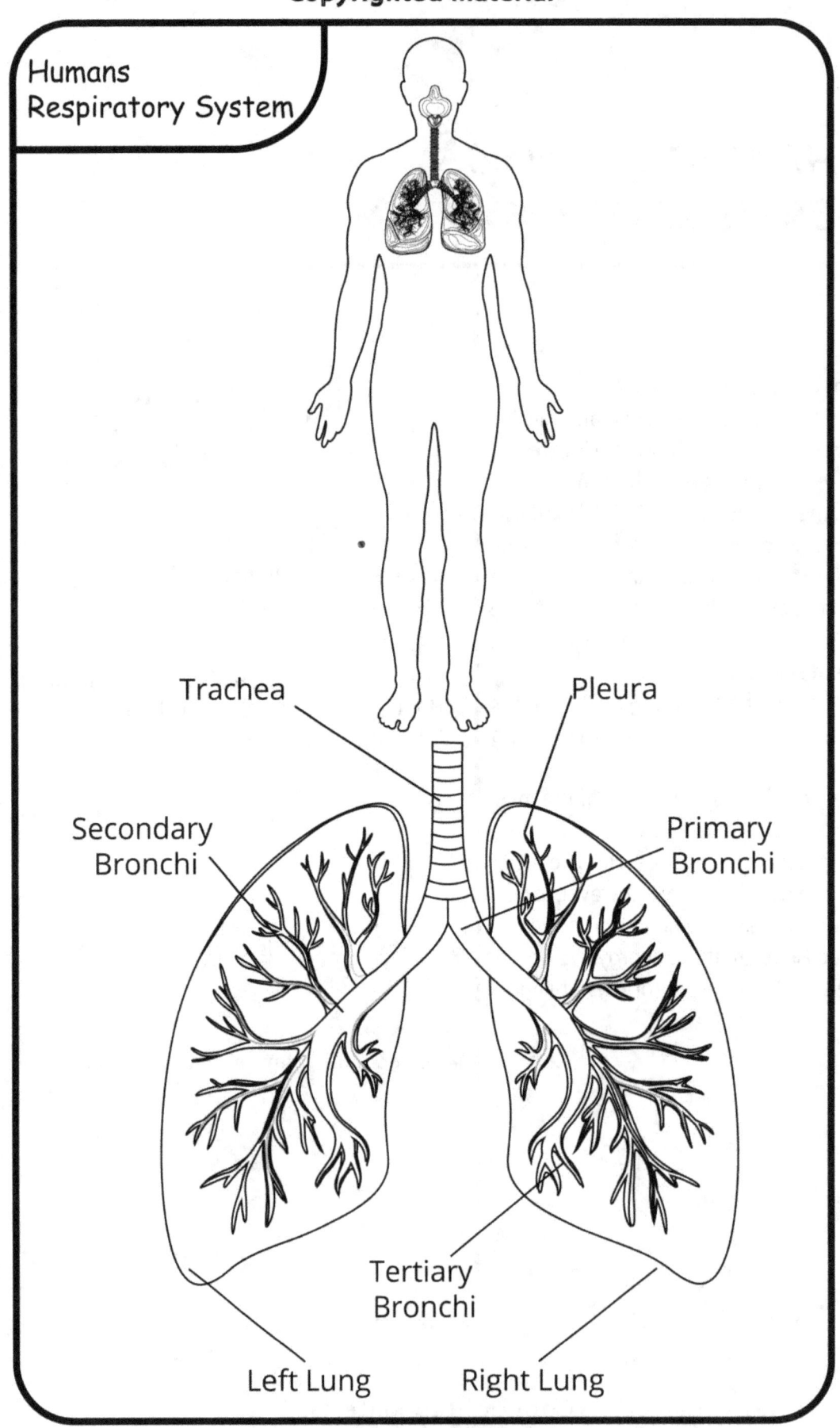

Trachea

Pleura

Secondary
Bronchi

Primary
Bronchi

Tertiary
Bronchi

Left Lung

Right Lung

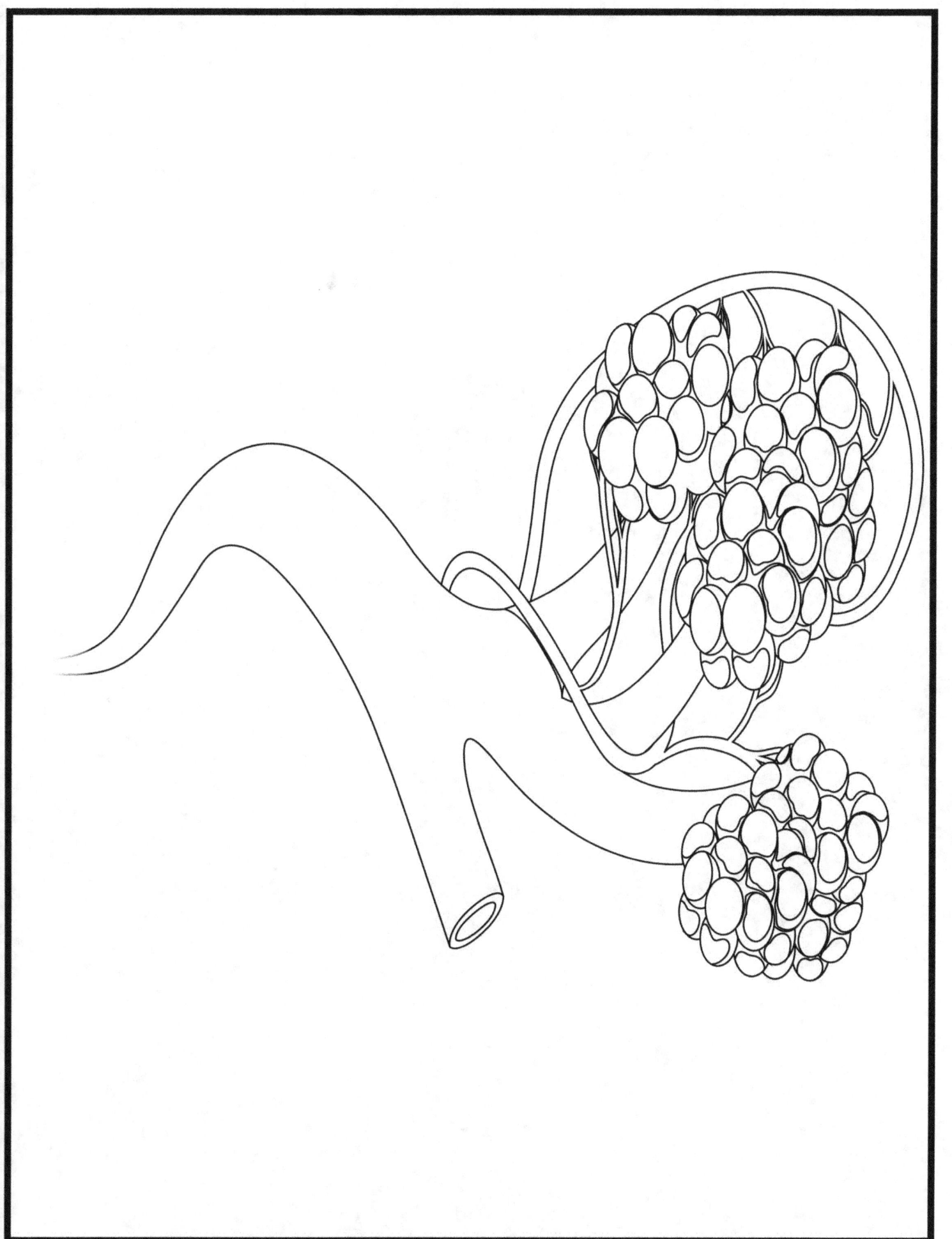

Color the organ below and put the right name :

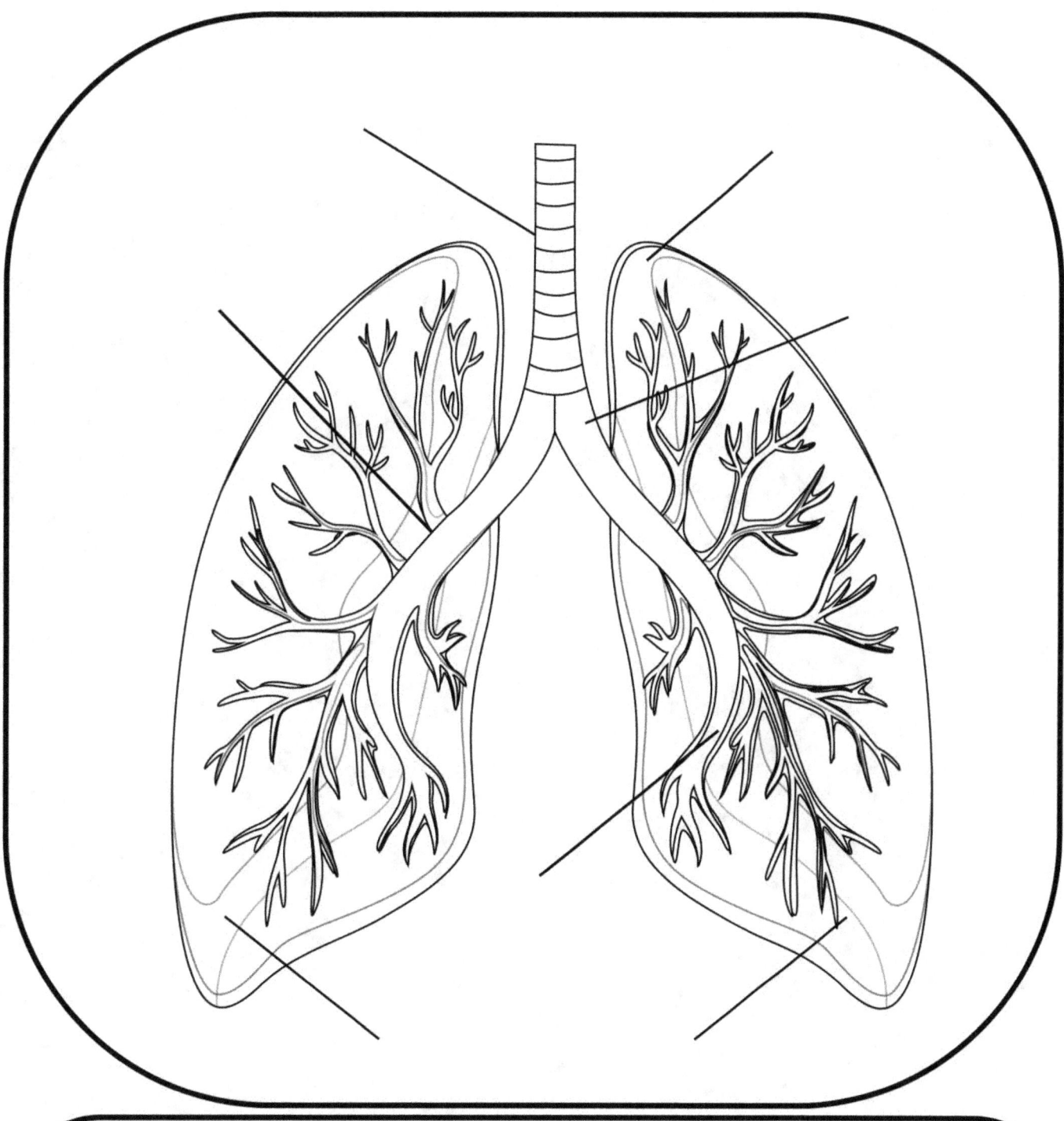

- Tertiary Bronchi / - right lung / - secondary bronchi / - trachea / - left lung / - pleaura

- primary bronch

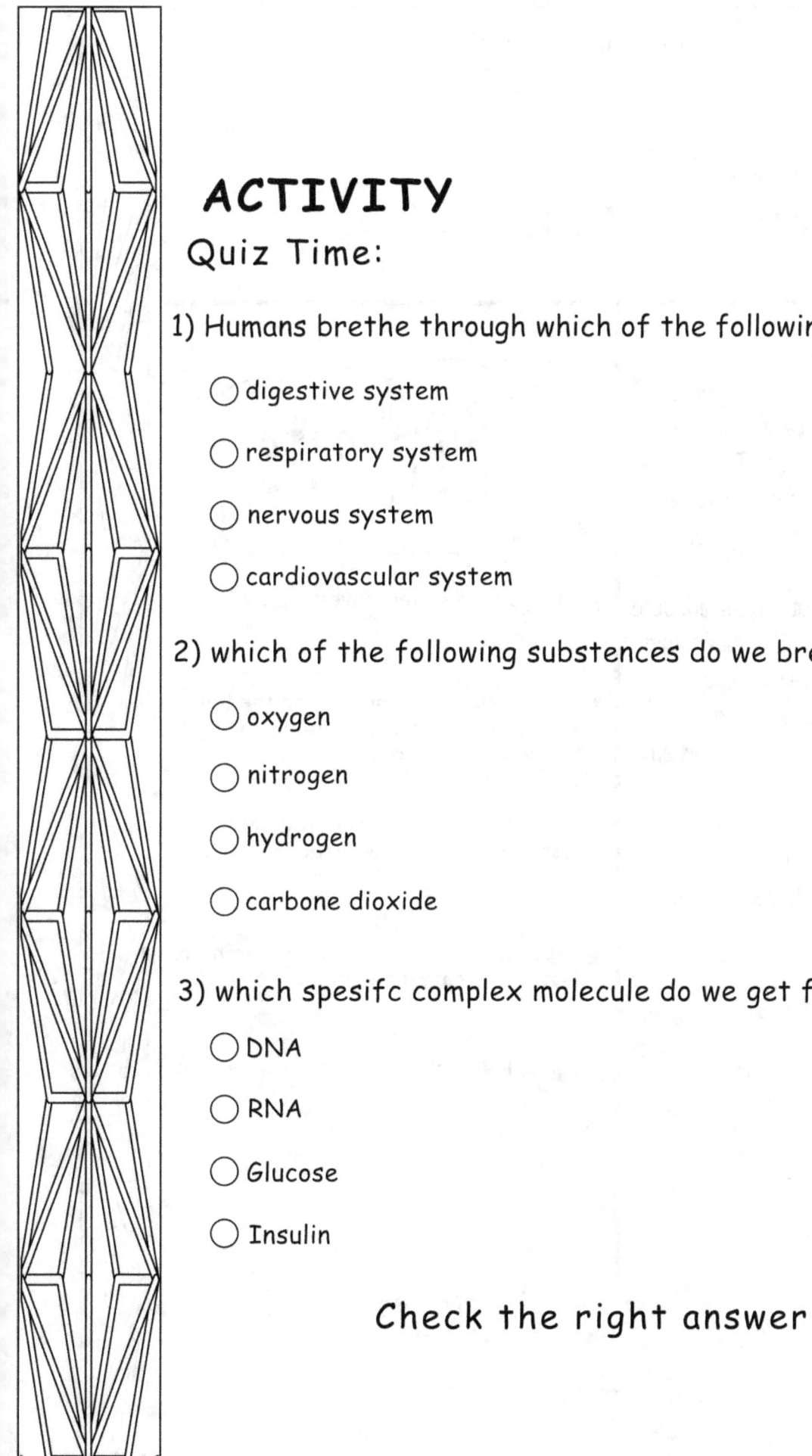

ACTIVITY

Quiz Time:

1) Humans brethe through which of the following systems?

○ digestive system

○ respiratory system

○ nervous system

○ cardiovascular system

2) which of the following substences do we breathe in ?

○ oxygen

○ nitrogen

○ hydrogen

○ carbone dioxide

3) which spesifc complex molecule do we get from eating ?

○ DNA

○ RNA

○ Glucose

○ Insulin

Check the right answer with (x)

SAFETY FIRST
OUR IMMUNE SYSTEM

The immune system helps to protect us against diseases caused by tiny invaders called pathogens such as viruses, bacteria, and parasites. The immune system is made up of specialized organs involved in the immune system include the spleen, lymph nodes thymus and bone marrow.

The immune system is very smart and can adapt to new infections. Our bodies gain immunities in two ways: active immunity and passive immunity.

Active immunity: when our bodies develop immunities over time through the immune system this is called active immunity.

Passive immunity: when we are born our bodies may already have some immunity babies get antibodies from their mother as they are growing in the womb.

Fun Facts

✦ The immune system saves lives.

✦ Before scientists understood the immune system, ilness was chalked up to unbalanced humors

✦ Two men who unraveled the immune system's functions were bitter rivals

✦ Specialized blood cells are the immune system's greatest weapen.

✦ The splean helps your immune system work.

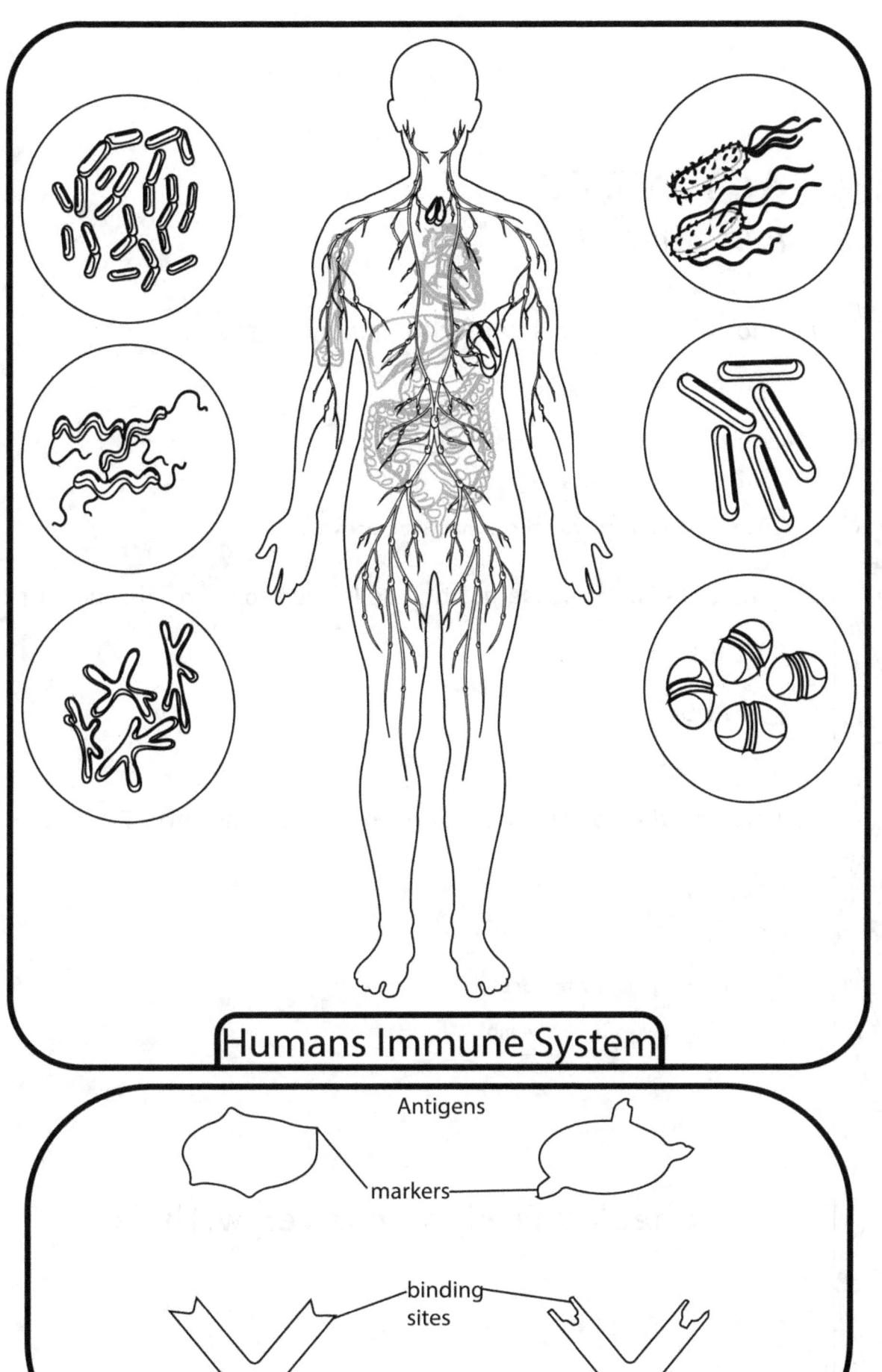

Humans Immune System

Antigens

markers

binding
sites

Antibodies

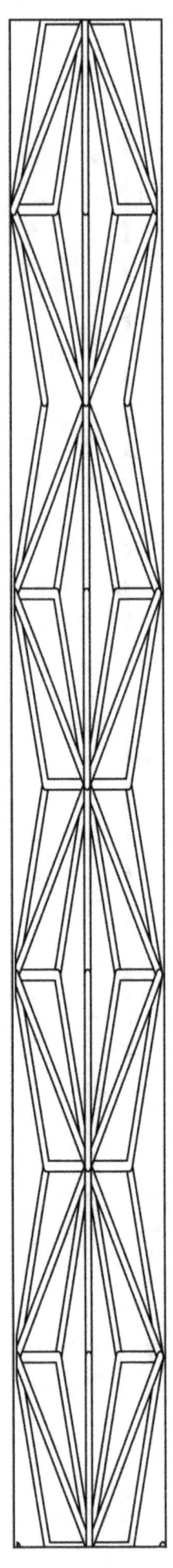

ACTIVITY
Quiz Time:

1) whats is the function of the immune system?

    ◯ to fight off diseases

    ◯ to break down food

    ◯ to regenerate cells

    ◯ to distribute energy throughout the body

2) True or False : disease fighting cells are stored all throughout the body

    ◯ TRUE

    ◯ FALSE

3) which of the following is not a way to get immunity ?

    ◯ vaccines

    ◯ nursing

    ◯ avoiding going to the doctor

    ◯ while growing in the womb

Check the right answer with (x)

take care of your body

Being physically healthy enables you to have better overall health, including in your relationships. You only get one body, so taking care of it is important. By knowing your body, and your family's health history, you can start to figure out what is normal for you.

Here are some tips fo taking care of your body :

◆ Eat a healthy, balenced diet with lots of vegetables and fruit.

◆ Keep your immunizations up-to-date.

◆ Don't use tobacco, vape products, alcohol, or drugs.

◆ Exercise as often as you can.

◆ Stay aware of your emotions and mood.

◆ Get enough sleep.

◆ Wear proper protection at home, work, or play.

◆ See your health-care provider if you think something may be wrong

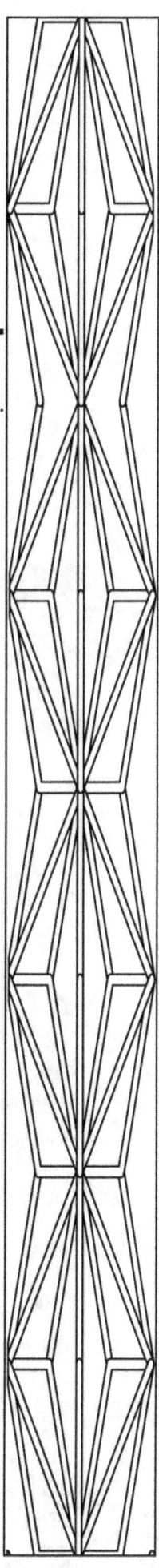